Introduction to
Human Neuroscience

Introduction to

Human Neuroscience

John A. Kiernan MB, ChB, PhD, DSc

Professor of Anatomy
The University of Western Ontario
London, Ontario, Canada

J.B. Lippincott Company Philadelphia

London   Mexico City   New York
St. Louis São Paulo   Sydney

Sponsoring Editor: Richard Winters
Manuscript Editor: Carol Florence
Indexer: J. A. Kiernan
Design Director: Tracy Baldwin
Designer: William Boehm
Production Manager: Kathleen P. Dunn
Production Coordinator: George V. Gordon
Compositor: TAPSCO, Inc.
Printer/Binder: R. R. Donnelley & Sons Company

Library of Congress Cataloging-in-Publication Data

Kiernan, J. A. (John Alan)
    Introduction to human neuroscience.

    Includes index.
    1. Neurobiology.   I. Title. [DNLM: 1. Nervous
System. WL 100 K475i]
    QP355.2.K54   1987   612.8   86-21330
    ISBN 0-397-50792-5

The author and publisher have exerted every effort to ensure that drug selection and dosage set forth in this text are in accord with current recommendations and practice at the time of publication. However, in view of ongoing research, changes in government regulations, and the constant flow of information relating to drug therapy and drug reactions, the reader is urged to check the package insert for each drug for any change in indications and dosage and for added warnings and precautions. This is particularly important when the recommended agent is a new or infrequently employed drug.

Preface

When students begin to study neuroscience, especially neuroanatomy, they almost always find the subject difficult. For most, the main causes of trouble are the abundance of new words to be understood, and the apparently unrelated facts that often take months to make sense. Over the years, many students have told me that they would like a short, basic textbook that could be read quickly at the start of a course, a book that gives them the significant facts in proper perspective and leaves out the details that can be learned later. "Introduction to Human Neuroscience" is an attempt to provide such a text. It is addressed primarily to medical students, but much of the material is relevant to some of the allied health sciences, such as physiotherapy, and to the nervous systems of animals other than man. The book may also be used for looking up facts that are required occasionally but are not worth committing to memory.

This text presents a brief account of the organization and functions of nervous tissue, with particular emphasis on the normal human nervous system. Many abnormalities are also described, for these reasons: (a) They provide the only clues indicating the normal functions of some parts of the human brain; (b) The correlation between the functional deficits and the pathological anatomy in some diseases serves to illustrate important facts of neuroanatomy; (c) Several neurological diseases (*e.g.,* stroke, epilepsy) are common enough to justify inclusion in any general text of neuroscience. Furthermore, the intelligent diagnosis and clinical management of these conditions demand a working knowledge of the relevant anatomy and physiology. Information of particular clinical interest is highlighted by the use of colored type.

Every school has its own way of teaching neuroscience; consequently, the order in which information is presented to students varies enormously. To allow for this, there are many short chapters in this book, each dealing with a single, clearly defined aspect of the nervous system. Although the chapters are in a logical sequence, the student can enter the text at any point selected by his instructors as the starting point for a given subject. Cross-references among chapters are frequent, and occasional repetition serves to highlight the information that is of greatest importance. Should the student encounter unfamiliar terms, he can locate their definitions easily by consulting the Index.

Most of the writing was done while I was on sabbatical leave in the Department of Anatomy and Cell Biology at the University of Sheffield, in England. I am grateful to Drs. R. W. Horobin and A. W. Rogers for making me welcome there, and also to the Commonwealth Scholarships Commission and the British Council, for providing a Commonwealth Medical Fellowship. Various illustrations and parts of the text have been constructively criticized by Dr. M. Berry of Guy's Hospital Medical School in London, and by Drs. A. J. Bower, I. N. C. Lawes, and M. A. Warren of Sheffield. Their kind help has resulted in several improvements. I wish also to acknowledge the expert assistance of Mrs. Maureen Tune with the preparation of the illustrations, and of Mrs. B. Cross, who typed the manuscript. The printed product is a testimonial to the work done by the staff of the J. B. Lippincott Company in the planning and production of the book.

J. A. Kiernan

London, Ontario
February, 1987

Contents

Chapter 1

The Nature and Organization
of the Nervous System

Multicellular animals higher on the ladder of life than the sponges all have nervous systems. A nervous system contains cells specialized for the rapid passing of signals within the animal's body. It coordinates the activity of the animal by controlling the contractile and secretory cells. The input to a nervous system comes from sensory receptors. These are cells or organs that can communicate physical or chemical events, inside or outside the body, to the cells of the nervous system. In all but the simplest animals, there are extensive connections within the nervous tissue. These encode patterns of signals that control purposeful movements, feeding, defensive and reproductive activity, and indeed the whole gamut of innate and learned behavior. Learning can occur because the intercellular circuitry of the nervous system continually adapts itself with use.

Neurons and Neuroglial Cells

Nervous systems range in complexity from the simple nerve net of *Hydra* to the mammalian nervous system consisting of brain, spinal cord, peripheral nerves, and ganglia. The conducting elements of nervous tissue are called **neurons.** Each neuron is a cell, usually with several long cytoplasmic processes along which the signals are carried. The nucleus and most of the synthetic machinery of the neuron are in the cell-body, or **soma,** from which the processes (**neurites**) radiate. A typical neuron has several short neurites, called **dendrites** (meaning little branches), that conduct principally towards the soma, and a single, longer neurite known as the **axon** (from the Greek for "axis"). The axon typically conducts signals away from the soma and has branches that touch the neurites of other cells. Each point of functional contact between neurons is a **synapse** (from the Greek verb "to join"). Nervous tissue also contains cells that do not carry signals. These are the **neuroglial cells,** often referred to collectively as "glia." They outnumber the neurons, with which they are intimately associated.

Communication Among Cells
Other Than Neurons

Nervous tissue serves the special function of communication, but there are other ways in which cells can exchange information. **Gap junctions** are regions of apposition of the surface membranes of cells. They occur in most embryonic tissues and in some adult tissues. Small molecules can pass freely from the cytoplasm of one cell to that of another across a gap junction. Thus gradients of concentration of developmentally significant compounds can exist across a mass of cells and may be important for growth and differentiation. Gap junctions between adjacent smooth muscle cells are important for synchronous contraction in many organs. Gap junctions also occur between certain neurons; they are called **electrical synapses,** and they permit coupled signalling activity of the cells. Most synapses, however, work by a chemical mechanism. **Endocrine** cells typically secrete hormones into the animal's circulation, and the hormones influence other cells without the necessity of close physical proximity. Non-neuronal cells may also influence each other by secreting substances into the extracellular space, but not into the general circulation. The use of short-range hormones in this way is known as **paracrine** secretion. Neurons often respond to circulating hormones, which thereby influence behavior. There are also neurons that release hormones into the circulation, a process termed **neurosecretion.**

Gray and White Matter

The somata of neurons are not randomly dispersed; they are collected into aggregations of tissue known as **gray matter,** from its color in preserved specimens. Gray matter contains cell-bodies of neurons, dendrites, and the beginning and end parts of axons. There are two main types of neuron. **Principal cells** have axons that leave the region and terminate in another region. **Interneurons,** which are smaller than principal cells, have axons that begin and end within the same region of gray matter. A circumscribed region of gray matter is a **nucleus.** A more or less isolated nodule containing neuronal somata is called a **ganglion.** (Some large nuclei in the brain are traditionally named "ganglia," though it would be simpler to confine this term to the peripheral nervous system.) Gray matter also forms extensive sheets of **cortex** (plural *cortices*) on some surfaces of the brain.

White matter is white from the myelin sheaths of axons, which are the principal components of the tissue. A **nerve** is a thread- or cordlike bundle of axons passing among organs made of non-nervous tissue. A **funiculus** (from Latin, "little rope") is a major bundle of myelinated fibers in the spinal cord. A **fasciculus** ("little bundle") is smaller. A **tract** is a population of fibers *en route* from one region to another; often a tract occupies a distinctive fasciculus. A **capsule** is a conspicuous sheet of white matter in the brain. Many axons cross the midline of the body. If they connect symmetrical structures, the crossing fibers constitute a **commissure.** A **decussation** is the site at which a tract connecting asymmetric structures crosses the midline. Axons coming to a region are **afferent.** Axons projecting from a region are **efferent** (Latin prefixes for "to" or "out of," respectively, with *ferre,* "to carry").

Structural Plan of the Nervous System

In man and in all other vertebrate animals, the nervous system has two divisions: the central nervous system is contained in the axial skeleton, and the peripheral nervous system is distributed through most of the other parts of the body (Fig. 1-1).

The Central Nervous System: Brain and Spinal Cord

The central nervous system is a hollow tube, the **neuraxis.** Its central cavity, the **neurocoele,** consists of the central canal of the spinal cord and the ventricular system of the brain. The structure of the neuraxis varies from place to

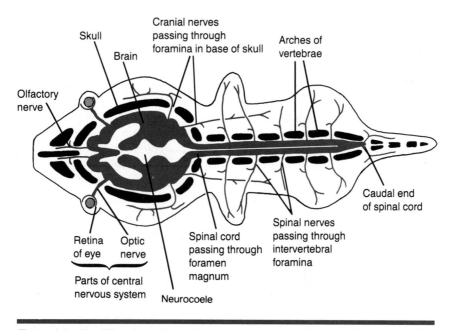

Figure 1-1 Simplified plan of the nervous system of a generalized vertebrate animal. The central nervous system, protected by the axial skeleton, is connected by nerves with all parts of the body.

place because of differences in the size and shape of the neurocoele and in the thickness of the wall of the tube. In higher animals, flexures of the neuraxis help to fit the essentially tubular brain into a round head. One end of the tube points towards the nose or beak (*rostrum*) and the other points towards the tail (*cauda*). Relative positions along the length of the central nervous system are defined by the terms **rostral** and **caudal.** These words are less ambiguous than the anatomical terms "superior," "inferior," "anterior," and "posterior." The **ventral** surface of the neuraxis faces the alimentary canal and the other internal organs; the **dorsal** surface faces in the opposite direction, towards the back and the top of the head. The **midline** is the plane that bisects the body, including the nervous system, into the left and right halves. Nearness to the midline is indicated by the word **medial,** whereas **lateral** denotes remoteness from the

midline. A **median** structure is within, or astride, the midline.

The rostral end of the central nervous system, contained in the cranium, is the **brain.** The caudal end of the brain continues into the **spinal cord.** This is contained in the spinal canal formed by the vertebrae and their connecting ligaments. The cranial cavity becomes continuous with the spinal canal through the foramen magnum, a large hole in the occipital bone. A **foramen** (from the Latin *forare,* to pierce) is a hole. Nerves connected with the brain or spinal cord pass through foramina in the base of the skull or between the vertebrae, respectively.

The spinal cord, like the vertebral column, is segmented, though the segments blend imperceptibly into each other. Left and right **spinal nerves,** one pair per segment, pass through the intervertebral foramina and are distributed to the trunk, appendages, and viscera. These nerves belong to the peripheral nervous system. There is an abrupt transition between central and peripheral nervous tissue at the surface of the cord. Equivalent junctions exist where the cranial nerves connect with the brain.

A segmented plan is not obvious in the brain, which is formed of three main parts, the hindbrain, the midbrain, and the forebrain. The **hindbrain,** which merges caudally with the spinal cord, consists of the **medulla oblongata** (usually called simply the medulla) caudally, and the **pons** rostrally. The **midbrain** (or **mesencephalon**) consists of the **tectum** dorsally and the two **cerebral peduncles** ventrally. The **forebrain** is the most rostral part of the brain. The caudal part of the forebrain is the **diencephalon;** the rostral part is the **telencephalon.** (These rather cumbersome terms are made up from Greek roots that mean "between-brain" and "end-brain," respectively.)

Dilatations of the neurocoele within the brain are called **ventricles.** The hindbrain contains the **fourth ventricle.** This is continuous caudally with the **central canal** of the spinal cord and rostrally with the **cerebral aqueduct,** which is the cavity of the midbrain. In the diencephalon the cavity becomes the **third ventricle.** Further rostrally the neurocoele bifurcates, so that the third ventricle leads into left and right **lateral ventricles.** Thus, the telencephalon consists of two **cerebral hemispheres,** each containing a lateral ventricle.

The neurocoele contains **cerebrospinal fluid.** This is secreted by **choroid plexus,** a vascular tissue that intrudes into the ventricles.

The shape of the brain is due partly to the ventricular system and partly to the variable thickness of the nervous tissue forming its walls. Some conspicuous and important parts of the central nervous system do not have central cavities continuous with the neurocoele, at least in adult life. The **cerebellum** is a large outgrowth of the dorsal and lateral surfaces of the hindbrain and midbrain. The optic nerve and the **retina** of the eye are outgrowths from the diencephalon. The diencephalon also has two glandular outgrowths: the **epiphysis** (or **pineal gland**) dorsally, and the **hypophysis** (or **pituitary gland**) ventrally. The **olfactory bulbs** are paired, stalked structures in the rostal part of the telencephalon. They are concerned with the sense of smell. The most conspicuous part of the human brain is the greatly convoluted **cerebral cortex,** which covers the surfaces of the cerebral hemispheres (Fig. 1-2).

The Peripheral Nervous System

The central nervous system is connected to other parts of the body by **nerves.** Neuronal cell-bodies outside the central nervous system occur in **ganglia** (singular, ganglion). The **spinal nerves** are segmentally organized. Each has a dorsal and a ventral **root,** separately connected with the spinal cord. The dorsal root bears a ganglion (called either a **spinal ganglion** or a **dorsal root ganglion**); the ventral root does not. The dorsal roots are exclusively sensory, whereas the ventral roots contain the axons of motor neurons and the axons of neurons controlling internal organs, blood vessels, and glands.

Paired **cranial nerves** connect the brain with other structures. The olfactory nerves, concerned with smell, enter the olfactory bulb, which is at the rostral end of the telencephalon. The optic nerves, like the retinas of the eyes, are made of central nervous tissue. Strictly speaking, therefore, they are not nerves but outgrowths of the brain. The remaining cranial nerves emerge from the **brain stem,** which consists of the midbrain and hindbrain.

Sensory and Effector Structures

The word **receptor** has two different meanings in neurobiology:

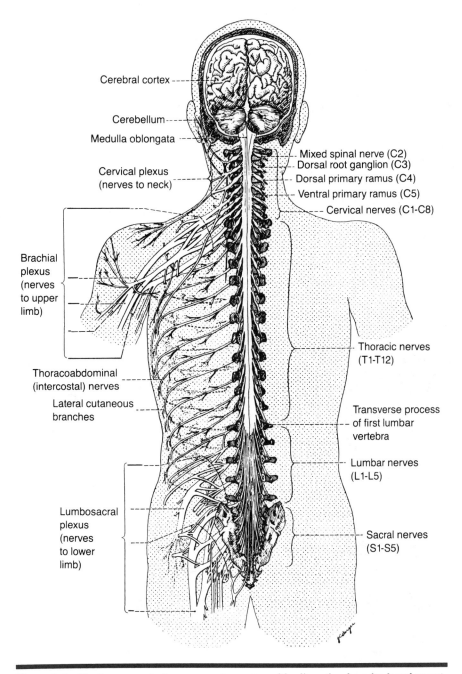

Cerebral cortex

Cerebellum

Medulla oblongata

Cervical plexus
(nerves to neck)

Brachial
plexus
(nerves
to upper
limb)

Thoracoabdominal
(intercostal) nerves

Lateral cutaneous
branches

Lumbosacral
plexus
(nerves
to lower
limb)

Mixed spinal nerve (C2)
Dorsal root ganglion (C3)
Dorsal primary ramus (C4)
Ventral primary ramus (C5)
Cervical nerves (C1-C8)

Thoracic nerves
(T1-T12)

Transverse process
of first lumbar
vertebra

Lumbar nerves
(L1-L5)

Sacral nerves
(S1-S5)

Figure 1-2 The human central nervous system, exposed by dissection from its dorsal aspect, showing brain, spinal cord, and the proximal parts of the spinal nerves. Compare with the generalized vertebrate plan (Fig. 1-1). (Copied with permission from Woodburne RT: Essentials of Human Anatomy, 6th ed. New York, Oxford University Press, 1978)

1. A macromolecule (on the surface of a cell, or sometimes inside a cell), which selectively binds molecules that initiate a response in the cell. Drugs, hormones, and the transmitter substances used for communication among neurons act upon cells by combining with receptor molecules.
2. A structure that acts as a sense organ, mediating conduction of signals into the nervous system.

An **effector** is an arrangement of contractile or secretory cells that either moves or secretes a product in response to activity in its afferent nerve.

Sensory Receptors. The simplest sensory receptors are the terminal branches of the axons of primary sensory neurons. The cell-bodies are in the ganglia of the dorsal spinal nerve roots and of cranial nerves. Free nerve endings are widely distributed in skin, blood vessels, viscera, connective tissue, and joints. Occasionally, as in hair follicles, there may be an ordered arrangement of the axons, but usually there is not obvious organization. Receptors of this kind respond to a wide variety of physical and chemical stimuli. Individually, however, they are specialized for particular sensations such as pain, temperature change, mechanical deformation, and the detection of substances in the extracellular fluid. The stimulus directly excites the surface membrane of the axon.

In structurally more complicated receptors, the axonal endings are associated with special cells that form a capsule, giving the sense or-

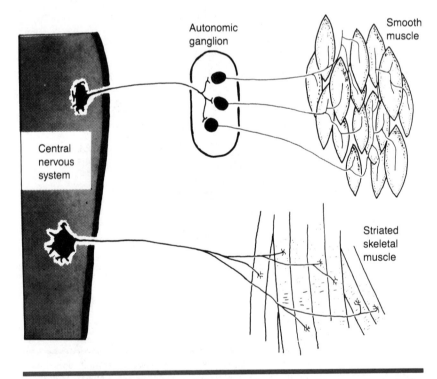

Figure 1-3 Skeletal striated muscle is innervated by neurons whose somata are in the brain stem or spinal cord. Smooth muscle is innervated by neurons of autonomic ganglia, so it is influenced, but not supplied, by the central nervous system.

gan a distinctive appearance under the microscope. These receptors usually detect non-injurious mechanical stimuli. The cells of the capsule may be involved in the process of **transduction,** which is the conversion of one form of energy into another. All receptors and effectors are transducers, and some of them can be validly compared to such inanimate electrical devices as the microphone, the television camera, and the electric motor.

Special receptors exist that generate neural signals from light, sound, position and movement of the head, and chemical stimuli in the mouth and nose. These sense organs all contain cells specialized for transduction, together with organized frameworks of supporting cells.

Movement and Secretion. The most conspicuous effector cells are **skeletal striated muscle fibers,** each consisting of a cytoplasmic tube containing many nuclei and a highly organized system of contractile filaments. The fibers are collected together to form **muscles,** which make up much of the bulk of the body. The ends of most muscles are attached, often through collagenous tendons, to the skeleton. Each skeletal muscle fiber is contacted by a branch of the axon of a motor neuron, whose cell-body is in either the brain stem or the spinal cord. A train of impulses in the motor axon stimulates the release of acetylcholine at the neuromuscular junction. The acetylcholine acts only briefly, because its destruction is catalyzed by an enzyme, acetylcholinesterase. Released acetylcholine triggers a series of changes in the muscle fiber leading to contraction. The coordination of the contractions of muscle fibers within different muscles results in purposeful movement. This coordination is a major function of the central nervous system.

The effector tissues in viscera are **smooth muscle, cardiac muscle** (only in the heart), and the **secretory cells** of glands. Some glands also contain contractile myoepithelial cells that serve to squeeze the secreted products into the ducts. Visceral effector cells are innervated by neurons whose cell-bodies lie in ganglia. The innervating neurons are themselves contacted by the axons of neurons whose somata are in the brain stem or spinal cord. Thus, a chain of at least two neurons is involved in the control of any visceral structure by the central nervous system. Figure 1-3 contrasts the modes of innervation of skeletal and visceral muscle.

Chapter 2

The Cells of Nervous Tissue:

Structural Aspects

This chapter and the next are concerned with the cell biology of normal nervous tissue. The constituent cells are described, and then the electrical and chemical mechanisms of signalling are explained. Most of the information in these two chapters applies to all nervous systems, including that of man. Much of the knowledge of neuronal function has been obtained from the nervous tissues of submammalian vertebrates and invertebrates.

The nervous system contains **neurons,** which are specialized for communication, and **neuroglial cells** (or **gliocytes**), which provide structural and metabolic support for the neurons. There is very little connective tissue in the central nervous system. Much more is present in the peripheral nervous system, because the nerves and ganglia are not protected by enclosure in the axial skeleton.

The central nervous system develops from an embryonic structure, the **neural tube,** and it remains hollow when fully grown. The peripheral nervous system develops from the paired **neural crests,** which are populations of cells that lie alongside the neural tube. All the neurons and gliocytes of the central nervous system are descendents of the cells that line the lumen (**neurocoele**) of the neural tube. Nearly all the neurons and gliocytes are produced before birth, but some neuroglial cells continue to be produced in adult animals, principally in a "subventricular zone" close to the lining of the neurocoele. The neural crest gives rise to the neurons and neuroglia of the peripheral nervous system.

Neuroglia

The word **neuroglia** means "nerve-glue" (from two Greek words); it is often shortened to **glia.** When the term was coined, it was thought that the tissue consisted of extracellular fibrillary and granular material in addition to cells. It is now known that the neuroglia consists entirely of cells, and that the fibrous and particulate elements are cytoplasmic organelles. The different types of neuroglial cells are described in Table 2-1 and illustrated in Figure 2-1.

The Neuron

As explained in Chapter 1, a neuron is a cell whose main function is rapid intercellular communication. Its characteristic features are a soma (or cell body) with long cytoplasmic processes (neurites = dendrites + axon) and points of functional intercellular contact (synapses). Rapid signalling occurs by means of electrical changes in the surface membrane

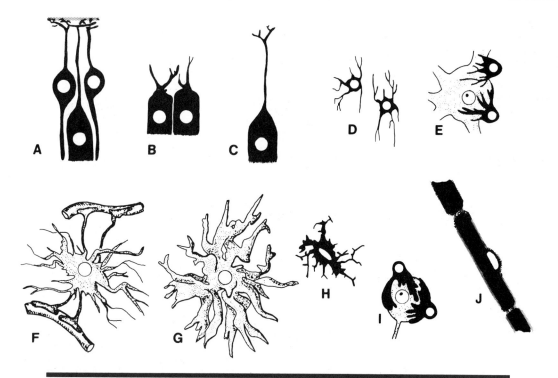

Figure 2-1 Types of neuroglial cells (see also Table 2-1). **(A) Radial neuroglia** (contacting the neurocoele below and the basal lamina of the outside surface of the central nervous system above. **(B) Ependymocytes. (C) Tanycyte. (D) Interfascicular oligodendrocytes. (E) Satellite oligodendrocytes. (F) Fibrous astrocyte** (with end-feet on capillaries). **(G) Protoplasmic (velate) astrocyte. (H) Resting microglial cell. (I) Satellite cells** with a unipolar neuron in a spinal ganglion. **(J)** Myelinated peripheral nerve fiber, showing one whole **neurolemmocyte** (Schwann cell) with a node at each end, invested by basal lamina (stippled).

of the neuron. Slower functions are mediated by the transport of many substances within the axon, both to and from the cell-body.

Types of Neuron

The shapes of some typical neurons are shown in Figure 2-2. There is great variety of shape and size, length of axon, and richness of branching of dendrites. Each type of cell, however, is fairly constant in its shape, and each type is found in its own anatomical site within the nervous system. It should be noted that in most types of neuron the dendrites

receive signals and the axon conducts them away from the region of the soma.

Generally speaking, there are two types of neurons: **Principal cells** have large somata and long axons that connect one region of the nervous system with another; **interneurons** have small somata and short axons (or occasionally no axon), and are confined to the region in which they occur.

Parts of the Neuron

The part of the neuron most important for the conduction and transmission of signals is

Table 2-1.   Neuroglial Cells

Name	Description

Gliocytes of the Central Nervous System

Radial Neuroglia

The first glial cells to appear in embryonic development. The nucleus is in the epithelium lining the neurocoele, and a long cytoplasmic process extends to the outside surface of the neural tube. Radial neuroglial cells persist into adult life in submammalian vertebrates. In mammals, they change into ependymocytes and astrocytes.

Ependymocytes

These form a columnar epithelium (the **ependyma**) that lines the neurocoele in the adult. Most ependymocytes have cilia. The basal surface of each cell has cytoplasmic processes that anchor it to the underlying nervous tissue. **Ependymal astrocytes** are cells with much-branched processes, in submammalian vertebrates. Ependymocytes with single, long basal cell processes are **tanycytes.** They occur in the third ventricle in mammals (Chaps. 26, 30). Special ependymal cells form the **choroidal ependyma** on the surfaces of the choroid plexuses, which produce the cerebrospinal fluid that fills the neurocoele (Chap. 30).

Astrocytes

The "star cells" have numerous processes. They are present everywhere in the brain and spinal cord. The cytoplasm contains glycogen granules and intermediate filaments (8–9 nm diameter) made of glial fibrillary acidic protein (**GFAP**). **Fibrous astrocytes** contain large quantities of this protein; they occur in tracts of nerve fibers and near the surface of the brain. Many of the cytoplasmic processes abut as **end-feet** on the basal laminae of capillary blood vessels. Astrocytic end-feet also form the thin **external glial limiting membrane** at the outside surface of the brain and spinal cord and around the larger blood vessels. There is a similar **internal glial limiting membrane**, subjacent to the ependyma. **Protoplasmic astrocytes** (also called velate astrocytes) have veil-like processes, which mingle with the tangled axons and dendrites of neurons. They contain less GFAP than fibrous astrocytes, and most of their processes are too thin to be resolved individually by light microscopy. **Pituicytes,** the glial cells of the neurohypophysis (Chap. 10) are atypical astrocytes.

At sites of injury, astrocytes enlarge and grow many new processes containing GFAP. They are then called **reactive astrocytes** (see Chap. 4).

Oligodendrocytes

The name means "cells with few branches." They have smaller, denser nuclei than astrocytes. The cytoplasm contains rough endoplasmic reticulum, polyribosomes and microtubules (25 nm diameter), but no glycogen or GFAP. Oligodendrocytes are conspicuous in rows between the bundles of nerve fibers: **interfascicular oligodendrocytes.** These cells form myelin in the central nervous system. **Satellite oligodendrocytes** occur, together with astrocytes, around the cell-bodies of large neurons.

Resting microglial cells

The rarest normal glial cells resemble oligodendrocytes, but are more irregularly shaped and have elongated rather than round nuclei. Once thought to be of mesodermal origin, they are now believed to originate from the ectoderm of the neural tube, as do the other glial cells of the central nervous system. Their function is unknown.

Reactive microglia

In injured or diseased central nervous tissue, these mesodermally derived phagocytic cells participate in inflammatory reactions. They are **monocytes** (a type of white blood cell), which have migrated through the walls of small vessels into the abnormal nervous tissue. (It was once thought that these cells were formed by proliferation of resting microglial cells, hence the name.)

Pericytes, cells adjacent to some capillary blood vessels in the normal brain, also are derived from monocytes.

(Continued)

Table 2-1. Neuroglial Cells *(Continued)*

Name	Description
Gliocytes of the Peripheral Nervous System	
Neurolemmocytes (Nearly always called **Schwann cells**)	These tube-shaped cells with elongated nuclei intimately ensheath all the axons in peripheral nerves. Each axon is suspended in the cytoplasm of its Schwann cell by a double layer of surface membrane, the **mesaxon.** The myelin sheaths of peripheral nerves are formed by Schwann cells. A myelinated axon is exposed to extracellular fluid at regular intervals along its length, where there are short gaps between adjacent neurolemmocytes. The gaps are called **nodes** (of Ranvier). One Schwann cell ensheaths either one myelinated axon or several unmyelinated axons. The surface of an unmyelinated axon is in contact with extracellular fluid along its whole length, through the cleft between the layers of its mesaxon. This cleft is closed off by the formation of a myelin sheath (see Fig. 2-4). On the outside surface of each Schwann cell, there is a basal lamina.
Ganglionic gliocytes (More often called **satellite cells**)	In sensory and autonomic ganglia, these cells intimately surround the neuronal somata. Ganglia also contain Schwann cells, around axons, and vascular connective tissue. The neuroglial cells of the enteric nervous system (Chap. 27) are derived from the neural crest, but these cells resemble astrocytes more closely than peripheral gliocytes. No special name has been given to the enteric glial cells.

(**Invertebrate animals** also have gliocytes. They are similar to astrocytes, and they intimately invest the neurons. The somata of the very large neurons of some invertebrates are deeply invaginated by glial cytoplasmic processes, which form a **trophospongium** ["feeding sponge"]. No invertebrate has myelin, but in arthropods several layers of glial cytoplasm often surround an axon.)

the **surface membrane,** or plasmalemma. The special properties of this membrane are discussed in Chapter 3.

The **nucleus** or a neuron is typically large and empty-looking. The chromatin is visible only as a darkly staining or electron-dense rim within the nuclear membrane, but there is a prominent nucleolus. Small neurons often have dense nuclei. The **cytoplasm** of the soma is dominated by the organelles of protein synthesis (rough endoplasmic reticulum and polyribosomes) and cellular respiration (mitochondria). There is also a well developed Golgi apparatus, where carbohydrate sidechains are added to protein molecules destined to enter or pass through the surface membrane of the cell. In light microscopy the rough endoplasmic reticulum is conspicuous as bodies of **Nissl substance,** named after Franz Nissl (1860–1919), a German psychiatrist. See Chapter 13 for a biographical note on Golgi.

Fibrous organelles are the most conspicuous components of the neurites. Microfilaments 4–5 nm in diameter, made of actin, occur on the inner surface of the cell membrane. They are also abundant in growth cones, which are the motile expanded tips of growing neurites. Intermediate filaments (9–10 nm) known as **neurofilaments** are most abundant in axons. Microtubules (24–25 nm external diameter) occur in all parts of the neuron; they are most conspicuous in dendrites and at the **axonal hillock.** The latter is the site on the soma, or on a large dendrite, from which the axon arises; it is also called the "initial segment" of the axon. Neurites also contain mitochondria and fragments of smooth endoplasmic reticulum (Fig. 2-3).

Dendrites taper with distance from the soma, and the diameters of successive branches become smaller. Synapses, to be described later in this chapter, are present over

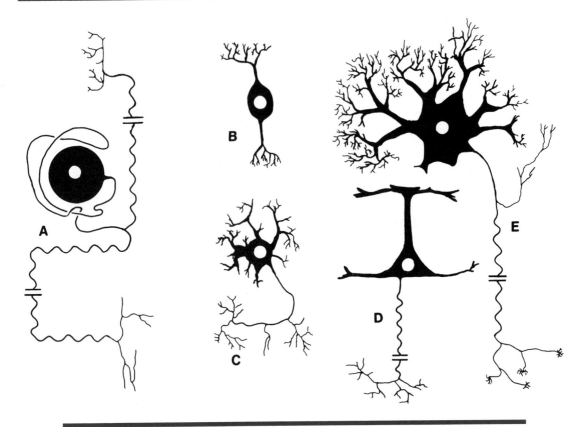

Figure 2-2   Some neurons, illustrating variation in shape and size. **(A) Unipolar neuron** of a sensory ganglion. **(B) Bipolar neuron. (C) Interneuron. (D) Pyramidal cell** (of cerebral cortex). **(E) Motor neuron.**

most of the surface of a dendrite. An axon has the same diameter along its whole length, and forms synapses in its preterminal and terminal portions. The axonal cytoplasm is called **axoplasm,** and the surface membrane is called the **axolemma.**

Myelin

Many axons are ensheathed in myelin. This is a close wrapping of many layers of double membrane derived from the ensheathing glial cell (see Fig. 2-4). The myelin sheath is formed by elongation and rolling of the mesaxon. The roll is so tight that the cytoplasm and extracellular fluid are squeezed out from between the layers of membrane. A Schwann* cell myelinates only one axon, but in the central nervous system each process of a single oligodendrocyte contributes to the myelination of a different axon.

The segment of an axon myelinated by a single Schwann cell or oligodendrocyte pro-

---

*Theodor Schwann (1810–1882), the German anatomist who described the neurolemmal cell, was also an originator of the "cell theory," which maintained that all organisms were composed of separate, living cells.

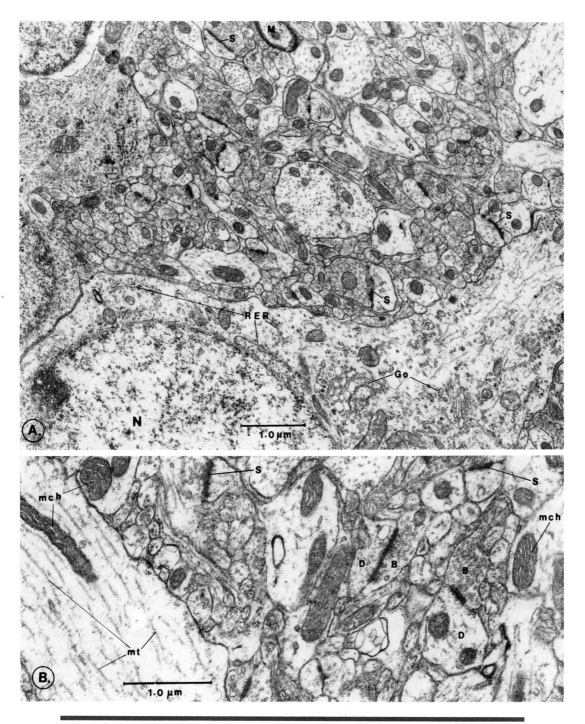

Figure 2-3 Electron micrographs of central nervous tissue (cerebral cortex of a rat): (B) Presynaptic bouton; (D) postsynaptic dendrite; (G) Golgi apparatus; (M) small myelinated axon; (mch) mitochondrion; (mt) microtubules (in a large dendrite); (N) nucleus of a large neuron; (RER) rough endoplasmic reticulum; (S) thickened membranes of chemical synapse. (Pictures kindly provided by Dr. M.A. Warren.)

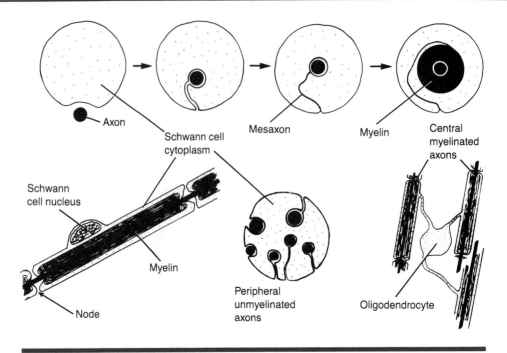

Figure 2-4 (*Above*) Development of the myelin sheath of an axon in a peripheral nerve, as seen in transverse section. (*Below, left*) Longitudinal section of a myelinated peripheral axon. (*Below, center*) Transverse section of a Schwann cell with unmyelinated axons. (*Below, right*) In central white matter, one oligodendrocyte produces the myelin sheaths of internodal segments of several axons.

cess is called an **internode.** Between the internodes are short interruptions (**nodes** of Ranvier[†]) in the continuity of the sheath. At these points the surface membrane of the axon, the axolemma, is in contact with the extracellular fluid. The electrical events of conduction occur at the nodes of a myelinated axon, and this provides for faster conduction of impulses than would be possible in an unmyelinated axon. Accordingly, myelinated axons occur in peripheral nerves and in the long tracts of the central nervous system. The unmyelinated axons in nerves are involved in functions for which great speed is not essential: some types of pain, and the innervation of blood vessels, glands, and internal organs.

[†] Louis Antoine Ranvier (1835–1922) was a French histologist and physician.

Nerve Fibers

A nerve fiber is an axon together with myelin sheath, if present, and the ensheathing glial cells. *The velocity of conduction of an impulse along a nerve fiber increases with the diameter.* The largest axons have the thickest myelin sheaths and, therefore, the greatest external diameters. The axonal diameter is approximately two thirds of the total external diameter of the fiber. The thinnest, most slowly conducting axons are unmyelinated.

In some invertebrates, notably annelids and cephalopods, there are unmyelinated axons 1 mm or more in diameter, known as **giant fibers.** These provide rapid conduction in animals that cannot form myelin, and they are involved in the control of movements that enable the animals to escape from danger. Cyclostomes (lampreys and hagfish) have no myelinated axons, but in their spinal cords are the large (50 μm) unmyelinated axons of the Müller cells, whose somata are in the hindbrain. All other vertebrates have myelinated axons for rapid conduction, so there is no need for unmyelinated fibers more than about 3 μm in diameter. Mauthner cells occur in the hindbrains of fishes and larval amphibians, one cell only on each side of the midline. Each of these huge neurons has a large axon that crosses the midline and then goes caudally in the spinal cord, to the neurons supplying the muscles of the tail. The Mauthner fibers are large, and in adult fishes they are myelinated. They are for stimulating fast, powerful movements used in escaping.

Table 2-2 shows the types of fiber found in peripheral nerves, classified according to di-

Table 2-2. Size and Conduction Velocity of Nerve Fibers

Name and function of type of fiber (letters are used for any nerve; roman numerals for sensory fibers in dorsal spinal roots)	External diameter (including myelin and neurolemma), in μm	Conduction velocity (meters per second*)
Myelinated Fibers		
Aα or Ia Motor to skeletal muscle; sensory from muscle spindle proprioceptive endings (annulospiral type)	12–20	70–120
Aβ: Ib Sensory from tendon receptors and Ruffini endings of skin	10–15	60–80
II Sensory from Meissner's and Pacinian corpuscles and similar endings in skin and connective tissue, from large hair follicles, and from muscle spindle proprioceptive endings (flower-spray type)	5–15	30–80
Aγ Motor to intrafusal fibers of muscle spindles	3–8	15–40
Aδ or III Sensory from small hair follicles, and from free nerve endings for pain and temperature sensations	2–5	10–30
B Preganglionic autonomic fibers	1–3	5–15
Unmyelinated Fibers		
C or IV Postganglionic autonomic fibers; sensory for pain and temperature	0.2–1.5	0.5–2.5
Müller fibers in spinal cord of lamprey	50	5
Giant fibers of squid (supply muscle of mantle)	1000	25

* At 37°C for types A, B, and C; at 20–24°C for the last two items in the table. The nerve fibers of cold-blooded vertebrates, corresponding to the mammalian types A, B, and C, conduct at approximately 1/3 of the velocities of mammalian fibers of the same size.

ameter and conduction velocity. Axons in the central nervous system are not as easy to classify; their diameters vary greatly.

Synapses

A point of functional contact between two neurons, or between a neuron and an effector cell, is a **synapse.** The structural details of synapses can be resolved only by electron microscopy.

Most synapses in vertebrate animals are **chemical synapses.** The surface membranes of the two cells are thickened by deposition of fibrillary material on the cytoplasmic sides. The intervening gap contains an electron-dense glycoprotein that is absent from the general extracellular space. The presynaptic

neurite, which is most often a branch of an axon, is known as a **bouton terminal** ("terminal button"; the plural is *boutons terminaux*), an old term that recalls the appearance in light microscopy. A bouton contains numerous mitochondria and a cluster of **synaptic vesicles.** The latter are membrane-bound organelles 40 to 150 nm in diameter. According to the type of bouton, the synaptic vesicles may be spherical or ellipsoidal, and they may or may not have electron-dense cores. More than one type of vesicle may be present in a single bouton. Synaptic vesicles contain the chemical neurotransmitters that are released into the synaptic cleft to act upon the postsynaptic membrane.

The postsynaptic structure is typically a dendrite. Often it bears a pendunculated pro-

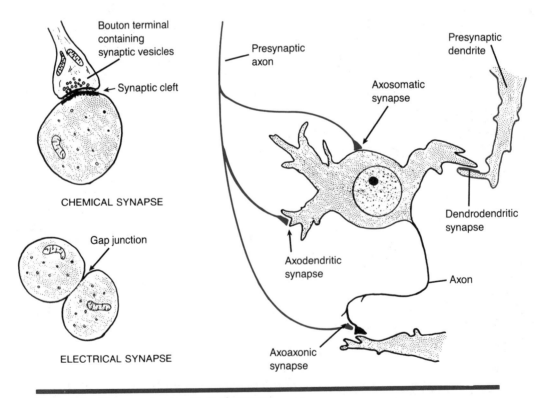

Figure 2-5 Diagrams of various kinds of synapses.

jection, a **dendritic spine,** that invaginates the presynaptic bouton. Commonly, synapses are grouped together on a dendrite or an axonal terminal to form a larger structure, known as **synaptic complex** or **glomerulus.** In the central nervous system, the cytoplasmic processes of protoplasmic astrocytes intimately invest synaptic complexes, probably to restrict diffusion of transmitters in the intercellular spaces.

Some different types of chemical synapse are shown in Figure 2-5. The most common arrangements for transferring signals from one neuron to another are axodendritic and axosomatic synapses. Axoaxonal synapses are strategically placed to interfere either with the initiation of impulses at the initial segments of other axons, or with the activities of other boutons terminaux. Dendrodendritic synapses can modify the postsynaptic responses to activity in other boutons.

The other type of functional contact between neurons is the **electrical synapse.** The cell membranes, usually of neuronal somata, are closely approximated (3 nm, in contrast to 25 nm for a chemical synapse). Large, tubular protein molecules bridge the cleft and are embedded in the surface membranes of both cells, providing channels through which inorganic ions, water, and other small molecules can pass. Thus an electrical change in one of the neurons is immediately propagated to the other, and the two cells are **electrotonically coupled.** The electrical synapse is identical to the gap junction or nexus found in many non-nervous tissues.

Chapter 3

The Cells of Nervous Tissue:

Functional Aspects

This chapter contains simplified explanations of the mechanisms of conduction of signals within and between neurons and the movements of substances within neuronal cytoplasm.

Membrane Potentials

The Neuronal Membrane

The surface membrane of a neuron, like that of any other cell, consists of a double layer of phospholipid molecules in which are embedded protein molecules. The special properties of the membrane proteins are responsible for the ability of the neuron to receive, conduct, and transmit electrically encoded signals. The most important membrane proteins are those known as "receptors," "channels," and "pumps." Receptors are discussed later in connection with synaptic transmission.

A **channel** is a tubular or ringlike molecule that permits the passage of inorganic ions such as sodium, potassium, calcium, or chloride. It is often a **gated channel,** which opens or closes in response to local electrical or chemical conditions. Ions diffuse passively through an open channel from the region of high concentration to the region of low concentration. A **pump** is a channel with associated enzymes; it consumes energy to move

ions from a dilute into a concentrated solution. The energy for this process comes from the hydrolysis of adenosine triphosphate (ATP), which is the universal source of energy in cells. The protein of which a pump is composed has enzymatic activity (ATPase) that catalyzes the hydrolysis of ATP.

Resting Membrane Potential

The most abundant ions in extracellular fluid are sodium (Na^+) and chloride (Cl^-). Inside the cell, potassium (K^+) is the main positive ion; it is neutralized by organic anions of amino acids and proteins. Both the extracellular fluid and the cytoplasm are electrically neutral, and each has the same total osmotic pressure. A consequence of these conditions is that there is a potential difference across the membrane: The inside is negative (-70 mV) with respect to the outside when the neuron is not conducting a signal. This **resting membrane potential** opposes the outward diffusion of K^+ and the inward diffusion of Cl^- because unlike charges attract, and like charges repel one another. The membrane is much less permeable to Na^+ because the voltage-gated channels for this cation are closed as a consequence of the resting membrane potential. The cytoplasmic anions are too big to pass through the membrane. The ionic concentrations are maintained by the activity of the **sodium pump.** This is a protein in the membrane that simultaneously expels sodium ions from the cytoplasm and withdraws potassium ions from the extracellular fluid. The sodium pump is also known as Na/K-ATPase.

Depolarization and Hyperpolarization

Neuronal signals are changes in the membrane potential that propagate over the surface of the cell and along the neurites. A stimulus initiating such a change is the combination of neurotransmitter molcules with receptors at a synapse on a dendrite. An excitatory stimulus causes reduction of the resting membrane potential from −70 mV to some lower (less negative) value. The change in potential spreads laterally in the membrane from its site of initiation. A sufficient number of excitatory stimuli will reduce the potential over the whole surface of the dendrites and soma. If at the axonal hillock the potential is lowered to a critical level of approximately −20 mV, it has the effect of opening the gated sodium channels there. Na$^+$ diffuses in and the membrane potential at the axonal hillock is immediately reversed to about +40 mV inside, a condition known as **depolarization.** A wave of depolarization, known as an **action potential** or **impulse,** will then be propagated along the axon in the manner to be described presently. In the laboratory, impulses may be initiated by direct electrical stimulation of nervous tissue. The size of the smallest stimulus that will trigger an action potential is the **threshold.**

An inhibitory stimulus causes the resting membrane potential to be increased to a value greater than −70 mV. This is **hyperpolarization.** Probably every neuron in the central nervous system receives both excitatory and inhibitory synapses. The more a postsynaptic neuron is hyperpolarized, the more excitatory stimuli will be needed to reduce the membrane potential at the axonal hillock to the threshold for initiation of an impulse.

Propagation of Impulses

In the dendrites and soma of a neuron, the changes in membrane potential are graded; they vary in time and space with the incoming synaptic activity. The axon, on the other hand, conducts impulses, which are waves of complete depolarization of the membrane, in an all-or-none fashion. Conduction in unmyelinated axons will be considered first. The physics and chemistry of conduction were discovered in the giant axons of the squid (see Table 2-2), which are easier to work with than the nerve fibers of vertebrates. The mechanisms are now known to be similar in all animals.

Consider a point on an axon before, during, and after the passage of an action potential. The following events occur:

1. The imminent arrival of the impulse causes a reduction of the membrane potential from about −70 to about −20 mV.
2. This amount of reduction in potential is the threshold for depolarization, and it opens the voltage-gated sodium channels. Sodium ions immediately move into the axoplasm. They do this because (a) they are attracted by the negative charge inside, and (b) the concentration of Na$^+$ outside is much higher than inside. The inrush of Na$^+$ causes reversal of the membrane potential to about +40 mV in less than 1 millisecond.
3. The sodium channels close, and the influx of Na$^+$ ceases. This is called **inactivation** of the channels. At the same time, the voltage-gated potassium channels open in response to the depolarization caused by the

incoming Na$^+$. Potassium ions now move out of the axon. They do so because (a) they are, at this moment, electrically repelled by the intra-axonal excess of positive charge due to the influx of Na$^+$, and (b) the concentration of K$^+$ inside is much higher than outside.

4. The outward diffusion of K$^+$ takes about 2 milliseconds to restore the membrane potential to its original -70 mV. The recovery is assisted by the sodium pumps, which expel Na$^+$ and pull in K$^+$. The membrane becomes slightly hyperpolarized (-80 mV) at this time, for about 1 millisecond.

5. While the membrane potential is being restored to the resting level of -70 mV, the sodium channels remain closed (inactivated), so the membrane cannot be depolarized. It is said to be **refractory.** The axon is refractory for about 2 milliseconds after the passage of an action potential; this prevents backward propagation of the impulse.

6. The depolarization due to influx of Na$^+$ spreads in both directions, lowering the membrane potential to the threshold value of about -20 mV. This change has no effect on the refractory membrane that is still recovering from the passage of the action potential. In the forward direction, however, the axonal membrane is not refractory, so reduction of the potential to -20 mV opens the gates of the sodium channels. There is a rapid influx of Na$^+$, and the membrane is depolarized.

7. The continuous repetition of this cycle of ionic movements results in propagation of the action potential in one direction. The events are shown graphically in Figure 3-1.

The ionic movements and resultant electrical changes are not the same in all neurons. Gated channels exist for ions other than Na$^+$ and K$^+$. **Calcium channels** have special significance in the presynaptic parts of axons. In the resting state, the concentration of Ca^{2+} is much lower in the axoplasm than in the extracellular fluid. When an action potential arrives, calcium channels open, and at presynaptic sites the influx of Ca^{2+} triggers the secretion of neurotransmitter molecules into the synaptic cleft. Calcium ions, like sodium ions, are removed from cytoplasm by an energy-consuming pumping mechanism.

Saltatory Conduction in Myelinated Axons

The velocity of conduction of an action potential along an unmyelinated axon increases in proportion to the square root of the diameter. Thus a mammalian unmyelinated fiber (0.2–1.5 μm) conducts at 0.5 to 2.5 meters per second, and a squid's giant axon (1.0 mm) conducts at about 25 meters per second. An advanced nervous system, which needs great numbers of rapidly conducting axons, would be impracticably large if it had to rely on unmyelinated nerve fibers.

Myelination allows very high conduction velocities (up to 120 meters per second) without an inordinate increase in diameter. In a myelinated axon, all the sodium and potassium channels are concentrated at the nodes. The internodes are electrically insulated by the layers of membrane that make up the myelin sheath. The myelin accounts for about one third of the total diameter of a nerve fiber, and the length of an internode is about 100 times the external diameter.

The ionic movements of an action potential can occur only at the nodes, but electrical conduction along the internodal axon, which behaves as a well-insulated wire, reduces the membrane potential to its threshold level at the next node. Thus the impulse jumps quickly from node to node. This form of prop-

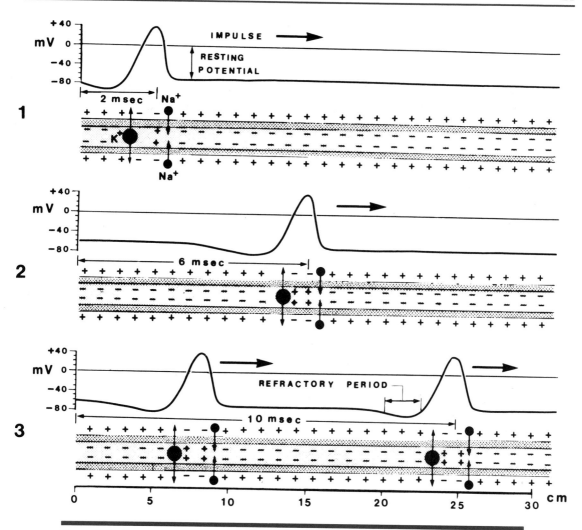

Figure 3-1   Propagation of an action potential (impulse) at 25 meters per second along an unmy-elinated giant axon of a squid. Localized influx of sodium ions (Na^+) is followed by an efflux of potassium ions (K^+) through channels that are "gated," or controlled, by voltage changes across the axolemma (**1**). The impulse begins with a slight depolarization, or reduction in the negative potential across the membrane, typically at the place where the axon leaves the neuronal cell-body. The initial voltage shift opens some of the sodium channels, shifting the voltage still further. The influx of Na^+ continues until the inside surface of the membrane is locally positive. This voltage reversal closes the sodium channels and opens the potassium channels. The efflux of K^+ quickly restores the negative membrane potential. The voltage reversal (action potential) propagates along the axon (**1, 2**) from its site of initiation. After a brief refractory period, a second impulse can follow (**3**). (Copied with permission from Stevens C: Propagation of the nerve impulse. Scientific American 241:54–65, 1979. Copyright© 1979 by Scientific American, Inc. All rights reserved.)

agation is called **saltatory conduction** (from the Latin *saltare,* to jump).

Conduction Velocity and the Compound Action Potential

The fibers in mammalian peripheral nerves are classified as in Table 2-2. Comparable populations of axons exist in the central nervous system, but are not included in any generally recognized system of classification. The letters A, B, and C, and the subtypes α, β, γ, and δ of group A, come from the phases of the **compound action potential.** This is a response recorded by an electrode in contact with a whole nerve. Following a brief electric shock at a distant point on the nerve, action potentials are initiated and propagated in all the axons. These impulses reach the recording electrode at different times, determined by the conduction velocities of the axons (Fig. 3-2).

It is possible to dissect successively thinner strands from a nerve until one is obtained that contains only a single functioning nerve fiber. The action potentials recorded from such individual fibers can be related to function. The Roman numerals used to name sensory fibers (see Table 2-2) were originally used in studies of single fibers dissected from dorsal spinal roots.

Postsynaptic Potentials: Excitation and Inhibition

At a chemical synapse, the arrival of an impulse at the presynaptic terminal depolarizes the membrane by opening sodium and calcium channels. The resultant entry of calcium ions induces release of the transmitter substance into the synaptic cleft. The transmitter molecules bind to **receptors** on the postsynaptic side of the cleft. The receptors are protein molecules with high specificity and affinity for the transmitter. Binding of transmitter to receptor affects the ion channels in the postsynaptic membrane. One of two things happens.

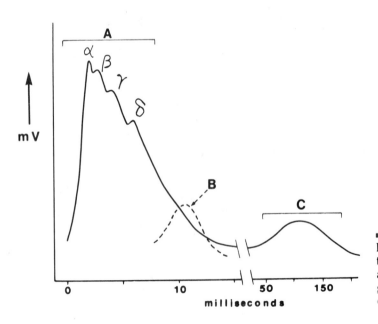

Figure 3-2   A compound action potential, as recorded from a nerve in a limb of any mammal. The B wave, due to preganglionic autonomic fibers, would not be recorded from such a nerve.

Either the sodium channels open, some Na^+ enters the cell, and the membrane potential is reduced (For example, it may fall from -70 to -60 mV.) This change is called an **excitatory postsynaptic potential (EPSP),** because a sufficient number of such potentials in a short time will add together and excite [depolarize] the neuron enough to initiate an action potential;

Or the potassium channels open, some K^+ leaves the cell, and the membrane potential is increased (For example, it may rise from -70 to -80 mV.) This change is called an **inhibitory postsynaptic potential (IPSP),** because the hyperpolarization of the membrane makes excitation more difficult to achieve. Some IPSPs are due to opening of chloride channels. The entry of Cl^- then hyperpolarizes the membrane.

The postsynaptic changes in membrane potential spread laterally over the surface of the cell by electrical conduction through the cytoplasm. The dendrites and soma of a neuron ordinarily receive many synapses of both excitatory and inhibitory types, so that EPSPs and IPSPs are constantly developing at many points on the surface of the cell. The two types of postsynaptic potential have opposing effects on the net membrane potential. If the potential at the axonal hillock is reduced to a threshold value, an all-or-none action potential is initiated and travels along the axon.

The efficacy of an individual synapse is determined by its distance from the site at which impulses are initiated. Thus, a small number of IPSPs produced near the axonal hillock can counteract the effect of a large number of EPSPs in the ends of the dendrites. Hyperpolarization in the dendrites and soma of a neuron is called **postsynaptic inhibition.** There are axo-axonal synapses that can arrest the propagation of impulses in the terminal parts of axons, preventing the depolarization of the boutons terminaux. Such synapses produce **presynaptic inhibition.**

Action potentials occur only in axons, so they give rise to EPSPs or IPSPs only at synapses where the presynaptic elements are axons. When the presynaptic neurite is not an axon, as in a dendro-dendritic synapse, the release of the substance is triggered by a smaller, slower depolarization of the membrane. The released transmitter evokes a postsynaptic potential, just as it would at an axo-dendritic synapse.

There are some neurons that never conduct action potentials. At the synapses of such cells, transmitters are released in response to smaller, slower reductions of membrane potential than those that occur in axons. For example, the photoreceptors of the vertebrate retina (see Chap. 18) have sodium channels that leak when it is dark. The resultant lowering of the membrane potential causes continuous release of the neurotransmitter, which excites the interneurons of the retina. Light makes the sodium channels of the photoreceptors close, causing hyperpolarization and cessation of release of the transmitter. The interneurons of the retina also exhibit only slow changes of membrane potential. So do some other small neurons such as the granule cells of the olfactory bulb (Chap. 14), whose only neurites are dendrites.

Neurotransmitters and Neuromodulators

It was once thought that a neuron used only one transmitter at all its synaptic boutons. It is now known that most neurons contain at least two or three substances potentially capable of being transmitters, and in many cases the appropriate receptor molecules are also known to be present at postsynaptic sites. This knowledge has been gained mainly by **immunohistochemistry,** a family of staining techniques based on the use of antibodies that bind specifically to the receptors, transmitters, or enzymes of transmitter metabolism. In only a few instances, however, has the occurrence of synaptic transmission by a known substance been proved beyond reasonable doubt. This is because the criteria for acceptance of a candidate transmitter are not easily satisfied. It must be shown that (a) the substance is present in the presynaptic parts of the neuron in adequate quantity; (b) appropriate enzymes for the synthesis of the transmitter are present in the same neuron; (c) the substance is released in functional quantities by depolarization of the presynaptic membrane; (d) local application of natural concentrations of the substance to the postsynaptic cell causes the same response as activity of the presynaptic neuron; (e) a mechanism exists for stopping the action of the transmitter (this usually involves an enzyme that catalyzes the chemical decomposition of the substance and the reabsorption into the presynaptic neurite of the substance itself or the products of its metabolism); and (f) specific receptors for the suspected transmitter are present on the postsynaptic membrane. Often drugs are available that compete specifically with the natural transmitter for binding to the receptors. Such drugs may mimic the transmitter's actions (**agonists**) or inhibit synaptic transmission by blocking the receptors (**antagonists** or **blockers**).

The action of a neurotransmitter on the postsynaptic membrane is the production of either an EPSP or an IPSP. The same transmitter will often produce both effects, though at different sites. This is because *the postsynaptic response is determined not by the identity of the neurotransmitter, but by a property of the receptors to which it binds.* Two examples will illustrate this point.

1. Acetylcholine, a transmitter at many synapses, causes contraction of skeletal striated muscle cells. This action is blocked by the curare alkaloids, but is un- affected by atropine. Acetylcholine also causes contraction of intestinal smooth muscle, but here the action is antagonized by atropine and unaffected by curare. In both instances there is no doubt that acetylcholine is the transmitter released by the axons that supply the muscle cells.

2. Noradrenaline is the transmitter used by most of the visceral (sympathetic) postganglionic neurons that supply blood vessels in skeletal muscle and skin. Because of different receptors, noradrenaline causes vasoconstriction in the skin and vasodilatation in muscle.

The physiological importance of the coexistence of two or more possible neurotransmitters in the same neuron is not yet known. It has been suggested there is only one true transmitter at a synapse, but its action may be influenced by the presence of other substances. A **neuromodulator** would not itself induce an EPSP or an IPSP, but it would change the properties of the postsynaptic membrane so that the response would not be the same as that evoked by the transmitter acting alone. Many of the peptides and some of the amines secreted by neurons are thought to be neuromodulatory agents, though some may also be true transmitters at other synapses.

Table 3-1 is a list of substances thought to be neurotransmitters or neuromodulators in vertebrates. The list is far from complete. Many of these substances are also present and active in the nervous systems of invertebrate animals.

Axoplasmic Transport

A simple calculation shows that even a small neuron has most of its cytoplasm in the neurites. A long axon accounts for over 99% of the volume of the cell. Almost all the neuron's DNA and RNA are in the soma, so it is necessary for synthesized proteins and other substances to be transported distally in the dendrites and axon. Most of the knowledge of such transport has come from the study of the movements of substances in the cytoplasm of axons, hence the term **axoplasmic transport.**

Velocities and Directions of Transport

Although axons are very narrow tubes, different substances move within them at different speeds, and even in different directions, at the same time. Transport away from the cell-body is **anterograde;** that towards the soma is **retrograde.** The largest amounts of material moved in an axon constitute the **slow component** of anterograde transport, moving at about 1 millimeter per day. The substances transported in the slow component are mostly structural proteins: tubulin (the subunits of microtubules), actin (for microfilaments), and the subunits of the neurofilament proteins. The **fast component** of anterograde axoplasmic transport moves at 400 mm per day in mammals and birds, or at 200 mm per day in cold-blooded vertebrates. Microtubules are involved in fast transport, which is prevented by the microtubule-disrupting drugs such as colchicine and vinblastine. Substances moved in the fast component are contained in particles such as mitochondria or small vesicles of the smooth endoplasmic reticulum. They include enzymes of neurotransmitter metabolism and peptides that are candidate transmitters or neuromodulators.

Retrograde axoplasmic transport occurs at about half the velocity of the fast anterograde component. Of the substances sent to the cell body, the most interesting are those that originate outside the neuron. Studies with radioactive and histochemically detectable tracers indicate that the presynaptic parts of an axon imbibe substances from the surrounding ex-

tracellular space. Such materials are then retrogradely transported to the soma, where they are sequestered in lysosomes and eventually degraded. Axonal uptake and retrograde transport provide a mechanism whereby the soma can receive information about the extracellular environment of remote parts of the cell by direct sampling.

Neuroanatomical Tracing Methods Based on Axoplasmic Transport

The axons and dendrites in the central nervous system are usually so closely interwoven that it is impossible to determine their exact sites of origin and termination by direct observation. Methods that label specific populations of neurons in experimental animals contribute greatly, therefore, to the acquisition of neuroanatomical knowledge. Such investigations are conducted in one of the following ways:

1. A radioactively labelled amino acid is injected into the region of the somata of a group of neurons. It is incorporated into proteins, some of which are transported anterogradely to the presynaptic axonal terminals. The appropriate parts of the brain or spinal cord are removed, after allowing time for rapid transport (often 24–48 hours), and prepared for autoradiography. The silver grains in the autoradiographs show the site of the injection, the axonal terminals, and often the trajectory of the intervening axons.
2. A histochemically demonstrable enzyme, horseradish peroxidase, is injected into the region to be studied. The enzyme may, with advantage, be chemically coupled to a lectin (carbohydrate-binding protein of plant origin). After 1 to 3 days, the distribution of the enzymes is examined histochemically. The sections reveal the cell-

Table 3-1.   Known and Suspected Neurotransmitters of Vertebrate Animals

Name	Chemistry	Some Functions
Acetylcholine (ACh)	A quaternary ammonium ion. Synthesized in bouton from choline and acetylcoenzyme A (choline acetyltransferase). Hydrolysis in synaptic cleft yields acetate and choline (acetylcholinesterase). Choline reabsorbed into bouton	Neurons using ACh are **cholinergic.** Known transmitter of motor neurons, all preganglionic and some postganglionic visceral neurons. Strong evidence for cholinergic neurons in several parts of brain
Dopamine (DA)	Primary amine, derivative of dihydroxyphenylalanine (DOPA). Formed by DOPA decarboxylase in presynaptic parts of axon. Reuptake by axon; also inactivation catalyzed by monoamine oxidase and catechol O-methyl transferase	Neurons using DA are **dopaminergic.** Transmitter in nigrostriatal pathway of mammalian brain (see Chap. 24). Also in many other neurons, including interneurons of autonomic ganglia
Noradrenaline (= norepinephrine or levarterenol) (NA or NE)	Primary amine formed from dopamine in presynaptic parts of axon (dopamine β-hydroxylase). Inactivation mechanisms, as for dopamine	Neurons using NA are **noradrenergic** (also often called "adrenergic"). Transmitter to most structures supplied by sympathetic ganglia (see Chap. 27). A hormone of the adrenal medulla. NA-containing neurons in brain stem (locus coeruleus) have axons that go to most parts of brain and spinal cord; probably modulates other synapses
Adrenaline (= epinephrine)	Secondary amine formed by N-methylation of noradrenaline. Inactivation probably as for dopamine and noradrenaline	Hormone of the adrenal medulla. Produced by some neurons in brain stem; significance uncertain
Serotonin (= 5-hydroxy-tryptamine) (5HT)	Primary amine derived from tryptophan (synthesis by a decarboxylase in axon). Inactivation by reuptake into bouton and by monoamine oxidase	Neurons using 5HT are **serotonergic.** Cells in midline of brain stem (raphe nuclei) have axons that send branches to most parts of brain and spinal cord. Raphespinal fibers inhibit transmission of pain signals (see Chap. 15)
Histamine	A heterocyclic amine derived from histidine (histidine decarboxylase). Several catabolic enzymes	Some evidence for excitatory function in the hypothalamus. Histamine from non-neural sources excites pain-sensitive axons in injured tissues, along with other mediators
γ-aminobutyrate (GABA)	Amino acid anion. Formed from glutamate by decarboxylation in bouton (glutamate decarboxylase). Uptake by postsynaptic cell and by neuroglia	Neurons using GABA are **GABAergic.** Always an inhibitory transmitter, in many parts of central nervous system including retina, spinal cord, and cerebellum
Glutamate and **aspartate**	Anions of common amino acids. Synthesis in neuron. Uptake by bouton from synaptic cleft	Excitatory action at synapses in most parts of the central nervous system. The two amino acids have similar physiological and pharmacological properties

(Continued)

Table 3-1.   Neurotransmitters of Vertebrate Animals (*Continued*)

Name	Chemistry	Some Functions
Glycine	Common amino acid. Synthesis in neuron. Uptake by bouton from synaptic cleft	Inhibitory action at some synapses in spinal cord
Adenosine triphosphate (ATP)	A purine nucleotide. It is released together with ACh, DA and NA, but may be the principal transmitter of some neurons. Several relevant metabolic pathways are recognized	Neurons thought to use ATP are said to be **purinergic** (an unfortunate term because the purine adenine is not a putative transmitter). Inhibitory to intestinal smooth muscle supplied by enteric nervous system (see Chap. 27); possibly also in the brain
Peptides (New neuropeptides are still being discovered. Only a few are listed here. Names bear little relevance to functions.)	Some are synthesized directly on ribosomes. Others are split off from larger precursor protein molecules. Catabolism rather slow, by proteolytic enzymes	Functions are all uncertain. Most peptides of nervous tissue also occur in alimentary tract, either in enteric neurons or in epithelial cells. Most neuropeptides occur in several parts of the nervous system. Sites listed below are not necessarily the most important ones
	Number of amino acids	
Carnosine	2	Olfactory bulb (excitatory) (see Chap. 14)
Thyrotrophin releasing hormone (TRH)	3	Hypothalamus (see Chap. 26)
Enkephalins (leu-ENK and met-ENK)	5	Brain stem, spinal cord. Transient morphine-like action on cells with opiate receptors
Oxytocin	8	Hypothalamus and neurohypophysis (see Chap. 26); hypothalamospinal fibers (Chap. 26, Chap. 27)
Vasopressin	8	Hypothalamus and neurohypophysis (see Chap. 26)
Luteinizing hormone releasing hormone (LHRH)	10	Hypothalamus (Chap. 26)
Substance P	11	Small neurons of dorsal root ganglia (excitatory); involved in axon reflex vasodilatation (see Chap. 13)
Somatostatin	13	Hypothalamus; enteric nervous system (inhibitory)
Vasoactive intestinal polypeptide (VIP)	28	Enteric nervous system (inhibitory); some autonomic ganglia
β-Endorphin	31	Adenohypophysis. Morphine like action on cells with opiate receptors; longer duration of action than enkephalins

bodies of neurons whose axons end in the site of injection, and also the axonal boutons terminaux of the neurons whose somata and dendrites were in the injected region. This method makes use of both anterograde and retrograde transport.

3. Different fluorescent dyes are injected at two different sites. After allowing 2 to 4 days for uptake by boutons and retrograde axoplasmic transport, sections of the tissue are examined by fluorescence microscopy. The somata sending axons to the two injected sites fluoresce in different colors. A neuron is labeled in both colors if its axon has branches that end in both the injected sites.

These methods can be used in all types of animals and are applicable to any part of the nervous system. They are the most accurate tracing methods available but cannot, of course, be used in human beings. Some other neuroanatomical methods are reviewed at the end of Chapter 4.

Chapter 4

Reactions of Nervous Tissue

to Injury and Disease

Previously normal neurons and neuroglial cells may change their behavior following any kind of physical, chemical, or infective insult. Common causes of disorder in the nervous system include direct injury, infarction (local death of tissue due to cessation of blood flow), hemorrhage, invasion by tumors, and inflammation (sometimes due to infection). In addition, there are diseases in which neurons or glial cells either die or fail to work properly for reasons that are not yet understood.

Any abnormality of structure or function in any organ is called a **lesion.** The localized death of part of an otherwise living animal is **necrosis.**

Gliosis

In non-nervous tissue, any space left behind by dead cells is occupied eventually by a **scar,** which consists largely of collagen fibers. Collagenous scars can form in the nervous system, too, but only when the lesion involves significant amounts of connective tissue. When a small part of the brain or spinal cord dies, the necrotic material is phagocytosed by **reactive microglial cells,** which emigrate from the blood vessels in the nearby living nervous tissue. The removal of the debris is much slower than in other tissues, and fragments of cytoplasm and of myelin can remain as extracellular objects for several months. The **astrocytes** adjacent to the necrotic site grow increased numbers of cytoplasmic processes, all packed with fibrils of GFAP (see Chap. 3). Sometimes the astrocytes may also increase their numbers by mitosis. The closely packed astrocytic processes eventually fill the abnormal area if it is small. In fishes and amphibians ependymal astrocytes, as well as ordinary astrocytes, contribute to the mass of glial cytoplasm.

If there is a large area of necrosis, the reactive astrocytes cannot fill it. Instead, they form a wall around the lesion. The middle of the dead area may eventually liquefy and form a **cyst.** If the damaged region touches the surface of the brain or spinal cord, there may be collagenous scarring from the surrounding meningeal connective tissue. Almost any kind of lesion in the central nervous system is associated with some necrosis. The subsequent replacement or walling off by reactive astrocytes is called **gliosis.** All scars contract with time. In the case of gliosis, the shrinkage is probably brought about by slow shortening of astrocytic processes, which pull on the surrounding blood vessels to which they are attached by end-feet.

All nervous tissue is delicate, but the mammalian spinal cord is peculiarly vulnerable.

After an injury such as compression by a fractured vertebra, the glial reaction continues for several weeks. Areas of cystic necrosis develop after the apparent healing of the lesion, and the tracts of axons in the cord can be transected by this delayed event. The final gliotic scar also contracts, so that the cord is narrowed greatly at the site of the original compression. It has been suggested that dense gliosis prevents regeneration of axons in the brain and spinal cord in reptiles, birds, and mammals. However, axons are able to grow through comparably dense glial scars in fishes and amphibians.

Demyelination

In some diseases, axons lose their myelin sheaths. The most common demyelinating disease of the human central nervous system is **multiple sclerosis,** in which small lesions are scattered throughout the central nervous system. The disease has an up-and-down clinical course, with symptoms that depend on the positions of the lesions. Its cause is unknown. Several diseases known as **neuropathies** cause demyelination in peripheral nerves.

Myelin sheaths are necessary for rapid conduction of impulses. Demyelinated axons cannot conduct because they have sodium channels only at the positions of their nodes. In the absence of the insulating layers of myelin, electric current cannot be conducted from one node to the next. Restoration of conduction along demyelinated segments of axons can occur as a result of *either* remyelination *or* the development of new sodium channels in the surface membranes of demyelinated axons. The former process is very slow; the latter process permits only slow conduction of impulses, as in unmyelinated nerve fibers. Probably both mechanisms contribute to functional recovery in multiple sclerosis and in neuropathies.

In animals, demyelination can be produced with certain toxic substances, such as acrylamide or diphtheria toxin, or by inducing an immune response to certain proteins of the myelin sheath. **Experimental allergic encephalomyelitis** is an autoimmune disease of the central nervous system produced by inoculating myelin basic protein, an identified component of central myelin. Phagocytic cells strip off the myelin in layers from the axons. The lesions of this disease are scattered, as are those of human multiple sclerosis. Immunization against a protein of peripheral myelin causes a neuropathy, **experimental allergic neuritis.** These artificial diseases have been much studied because of their similarities to human demyelinating diseases.

Effects of Axonal Transection

The part of an axon that has been separated from its cell-body is able to conduct impulses for a few days before it dies. The whole nerve fiber then breaks into fragments. The axon and its myelin sheath disintegrate, even though the latter is not part of the neuron. Eventually the fragments are phagocytosed, either promptly by Schwann cells in a nerve, or slowly by reactive microglial cells in the central nervous system. The fragmentation and dissolution of the distal parts of a severed nerve fiber is called **Wallerian degeneration** (after AV Waller, 1816–1870, an English physician and physiologist who described the changes in transected peripheral nerves).

The soma of the neuron also reacts to axonal transection. The **axon reaction** of the soma includes swelling, a change in distribution of cytoplasmic RNA (**chromatolysis**), and displacement of the nucleus from the center to the edge of the cell. These events are associated with increased synthesis of proteins. Later changes in the soma depend on events at the site of transection. If the axon regenerates (see below), the appearance returns slowly to normal. If axonal regeneration does not occur, the cell-body shrinks and eventually may die. The axon reaction is seen when a substantial portion of cytoplasm has been removed. It is often undetectable when only one branch of an axon has been cut.

Occasionally, axonal transection causes degenerative changes in the somata of other neurons, those with which the lost axon synapsed. This is **transneuronal degeneration,** which occurs, for example, in the mammalian visual system. Transection of an optic tract is followed by chromatolysis in the lateral geniculate body.

Successful Axonal Regeneration

It is important to note that axonal regeneration is the replacement of a cell's amputated cytoplasmic process. It should not be confused with axonal growth that occurs in normal development, or with the abnormal sprouting of new branches from axons that have not been injured.

Peripheral Nerves

In all vertebrates, including man, the axons in nerves regenerate well unless there is considerable collagenous scarring at the site of injury. A few days after the axon has been cut, many thin branches grow out from its proximal stump. Distal to the site of transection, one of these sprouts enters a tube formed by the basal lamina of a series of Schwann cells. The other sprouts are reabsorbed into the growing axonal tip. The tube is filled by Schwann cells, which may still contain phagocytosed debris of the degenerated axon. Within the tube, the regenerating axon

lengthens in the cleft between the Schwann cells and their basal lamina. The tube guides the regrowing axon to preterminal branching points and then to terminations, such as neuromuscular or sensory endings. The rate of advancement of the tips of regenerating axons is 2 to 3 mm per day in mammals, or less than half that speed in cold-blooded animals.

The accuracy of axonal regeneration depends on the initial invasion of an appropriate Schwann cell tube distal to the lesion. If large numbers of axons are directed to inappropriate places, the functional recovery will be poor. The best results follow crushing or freezing. These injuries sever the axons but preserve the basal laminae of the neurolemmocytes and the connective tissue of the endoneurium. A transected nerve may be repaired with great skill, but the alignment of the tubes of Schwann cells can never be perfectly accurate. Axons that fail to enter the distal stump may stray into other nerves, or they may go on growing locally and form a **neuroma.** This is tender lump that can cause episodes of severe pain (**causalgia**), perceived as being in the area normally supplied by the nerve. The sensation of a "phantom limb" following amputation has a similar origin.

Having grown alongside the Schwann cells, the regenerated axon then sinks into the glial cytoplasm, forming a mesaxon. If the axon is one that should be myelinated, it induces the Schwann cell to produce a myelin sheath. Myelination or nonmyelination is dictated by the neuron, not by the neuroglial cell. Myelination of the regenerated axon and restoration of the diameter of the nerve fiber take several months for completion.

Some amphibians can replace amputated limbs. The development of the new limb is dependent upon the entry of axons into the initially undifferentiated blastema, the mass of cells that forms at the site of amputation. This is an example of a **trophic effect** of neurons on non-nervous tissue.

Central Nervous Systems of Lower Vertebrates

The axons of the optic nerve, which is part of the brain, regenerate efficiently in all fishes and amphibians. It is remarkable that the regrowing fibers navigate to the correct places in the tectum of the midbrain, and behavior requiring accurate visual connections is restored. In the optic nerve there are no channels comparable to Schwann cell tubes, and the mechanism of guidance of the elongating axons is not understood. Specific chemical affinities between touching cells may be involved. Axons regenerate across transections of the spinal cord in cyclostomes, fishes, and urodele amphibians (newts and salamanders). They fail to do so in anurans (frogs, toads), possibly because they are deflected by a collagenous scar. Axonal regeneration has been described in other parts of the central nervous system of fishes and amphibians, but has not been studied intensively.

Most axons cannot regenerate across sites of transection in any part of the central nervous system in reptiles, birds, or mammals. In some lizards, axons enter a short extension of the spinal cord that grows into the regenerating tail. Lizards' tails detach easily when pulled and then are regenerated.

Failure of Axonal Regeneration in the Mammalian Central Nervous System

Some axons do regenerate after transection in the brains of adult mammals. These are:

1. The neurosecretory axons in the neurohypophysis
2. Certain unmyelinated axons that contain amines (dopamine, noradrenaline, serotonin) as their suspected neurotransmitters

3. Axons growing into some non-nervous tissues that have been transplanted into the brain
4. Axons in certain tracts in very young rodents. This true regeneration should not be confused with the primary growth of new axons across a site of injury. Newly growing fibers are not regenerating
5. Axonal regeneration may occur *around,* but not through, small lesions that partly transect tracts of myelinated axons in the brains of rodents. Despite these occurrences, axonal regeneration in the mammalian central nervous system does not result in useful functional recovery, at least in adult animals.

Several hypotheses have been advanced to account for the failure of axonal regeneration in the mammalian brain and spinal cord. One widely held view is that mammals lack certain chemical factors which, in lower vertebrates, promote the regrowth of cut axons. Appropriate axonal growth factors might be secreted by neuroglial cells or they might circulate in the blood.

Axonal Sprouting

When postsynaptic cells have been partly denervated, there is often new growth of branches from the surviving afferent axons, which have not been injured. The new branches then form synaptic contacts with the denervated parts of the postsynaptic cells. This production of new, abnormal synapses has been studied in the brain and spinal cord, and also in muscle and skin. It has been termed "axonal sprouting," "synaptic replacement," and "plasticity." The first two terms describe the events observed; the third term has functional connotations that may not be justifiable. Certainly it is tempting to invoke axonal sprouting as a major mechanism of functional recovery from destructive lesions in the central nervous system. Infarction or injury of the human brain is followed usually by some recovery of function. With small lesions, the initial disability may disappear completely after a few months.

Axonal sprouting may be induced by chemical agents secreted by denervated cells. It is also possible that innervated cells produce substances that inhibit axonal growth. There are limits to the extent of axonal sprouting; an axon will not send new branches into regions other than those in which it normally terminates. "Regions" in this context may be delimited by neuroglial cells. In immature animals, such as fetal or newborn rodents, axons can sprout over longer distances than in adults, and it is possible to induce the formation of grossly abnormal tracts in the central nervous system.

Transplantation of Nervous Tissue

Nerve Grafts

If a long segment of a nerve has been destroyed, the only available surgical treatment is the insertion of a graft, which is taken from a less important nerve. The original function of the transplanted piece of nerve is irrelevant to its use as a conduit for regenerating axons, and it does not matter if the graft is inserted the wrong way around. Axons growing through a nerve graft meet obstacles at both ends of the transplanted segment and also are likely to be misdirected by the pattern of bundles of Schwann cells within the graft. The functional result is therefore less satisfactory than that following a simple repair.

Nerve grafts are taken from the same individual (autografts). A graft from another individual of the same species (allograft or homograft) is rejected. Therapeutic measures to prevent rejection of foreign nerve grafts are effective in laboratory animals, but are unlikely to be needed in clinical practice.

Grafts of Central Nervous Tissue

Adult central nervous tissue does not survive transplantation, even in the same animal. However, small pieces of brain from fetal rodents can be transplanted either into other fetal animals or into adults of the same species. Axons grow from the host's brain into the grafted tissue and, in some circumstances, axons grow out of the graft into the brain of the host. Axons can also grow into intracerebrally transplanted peripheral nerve, or into non-nervous tissue such as skin. If a peripheral nerve graft is used as a bridge across a site of transection of the spinal cord, some axons grow into and along the graft, but very few are then able to enter the central nervous tissue of the spinal cord.

Allografts placed in the brain often are not rejected, possibly because of the absence of lymphatic drainage. Antigens must reach lymph nodes in order to initiate immune responses.

Tracing Pathways by Observing Degeneration

The products of Wallerian degeneration can be demonstrated histologically with special staining techniques. Thus, if a tract of the central nervous system is transected, or if a group of neuronal somata is destroyed, it is possible to follow the courses of the degenerating axons to their regions of termination. The **silver methods** for degenerating axons in experimental animals have been rendered almost obsolete by the tracing methods based on axoplasmic transport described at the end of Chapter 3. **Electron microscopy** is valuable for showing the exact sites of degenerating presynaptic boutons. With any tracing method based on axonal degeneration, the investigator can never be sure that the lesion has destroyed only the intended cells or fibers.

The **Marchi method** (named after its inventor, Vittorio Marchi, 1851–1908, an Italian histologist), which demonstrates degeneration of myelin sheaths, is blatantly imprecise but still valuable for human material, because the stainable products persist for a long time. Fibers cannot be traced to their exact sites of termination with this method, because axons lose their myelin sheaths before they divide into their preterminal branches. The duration of human neurological disease rarely coincides with the critical time of 4 to 10 days needed for the more precise demonstration of axonal degeneration with the silver methods.

Chromatolysis, or degeneration, in neuronal somata can reveal the origin of a severed tract or nerve or the cells that innervated a destroyed terminal field. The changes are often difficult to recognize, however, and this experimental approach has been supplanted by methods based on retrograde axonal transport. Transneuronal degeneration occasionally has aided the tracing of functional sequences of neurons, especially in very young animals.

Chapter 5

Embryology of the Human Nervous System

Neurons and neuroglial cells are the descendents of certain cells of the embryonic ectoderm.

Early Stages in Development

Neural Tube

When the embryo has become three-layered, on about the 20th day after fertilization, a line of ectodermal cells in and near the midline thickens to become the **neuroectoderm.** The thickness is greater than that of the ordinary ectoderm because the neuroectodermal cells are columnar rather than cuboidal. The median part of the neuroectoderm remains close to the developing notochord, while the growth of the mesoderm on either side of the midline causes the lateral margins of the neuroectoderm to be more dorsally situated, as the **neural folds.** Thus, a **neural groove** is formed along the length of the dorsal surface of the embryo. The groove deepens, and the neural folds come into contact with one another and fuse, so that a **neural tube** is formed. The fusion occurs first in the middle part of the neural groove, destined to become the lower cervical segments of the spinal cord, on about the 22nd day after fertilization. Fusion of the neural groove proceeds rostrally and caudally (Fig. 5-1). The neural tube sinks into the mesoderm,

and the continuity of the ordinary ectoderm, which will become the epidermis, is restored. The holes at the ends of the neural tube are the rostral ("anterior") and caudal ("posterior") **neuropores.** In man, the rostral neuropore is closed off by continued growth of the neuroectoderm on the 24th day after fertilization. The caudal neuropore closes on the 27th day.

The neural tube will become the central nervous system. The site of closure of the rostral neuropore is represented in the adult brain by the lamina terminalis, in the rostral wall of the third ventricle. The site of closure of the caudal neuropore corresponds to the upper lumbar level of the spinal cord. The central canal of the lower spinal segments is formed by fusion of holes that develop in the mass of neuroectodermal cells constituting the caudalmost part of the developing central nervous system. The growth of the rostral end of the neural tube to form the brain is described later in this chapter.

Neural Crest

Some of the cells of the neural folds are left behind near the dorsal surface of the embryo when the neural groove closes to form the tube. These cells constitute the **neural crest.**

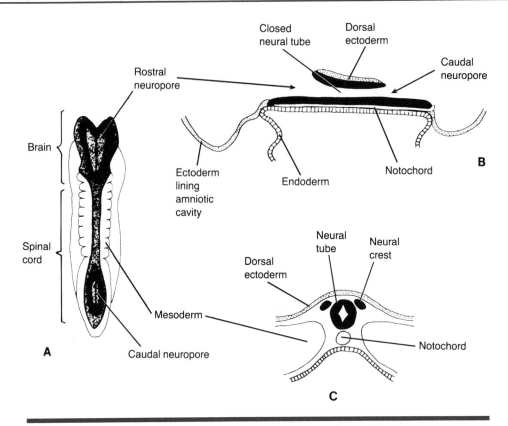

Figure 5-1   A human embryo 21 days after fertilization. **(A)** Dorsal view. **(B)** Longitudinal section. **(C)** Transverse section.

They proliferate and migrate extensively through the mesoderm, giving rise to the neurons and glial cells of the peripheral nervous system and to several other tissues. Nonneural derivatives of the neural crest include melanocytes of the skin, various endocrine cells, and some of the bones and other mesodermally formed structures of the head, including, probably, the leptomeninges (see Chap. 28). The morphogenetic movements that produce the neural tube and neural crest are summarized in Fig. 5-2.

Placodes

A few parts of the peripheral nervous system are derived from **placodes,** which are localized thickenings of the ectoderm in the head region. Thus the olfactory epithelium develops from an olfactory placode, and placodes also give rise to some of the neurons in the sensory ganglia of cranial nerves V, VII, IX, and X. Other placodes form the lens of the eye and the sensory epithelium and associated neurons of the inner ear.

Formation of the Brain and Spinal Cord

Histogenesis

The wall of the neural tube has three layers. The **ventricular layer** is next to the lumen, and all mitoses occur in this layer. External to the

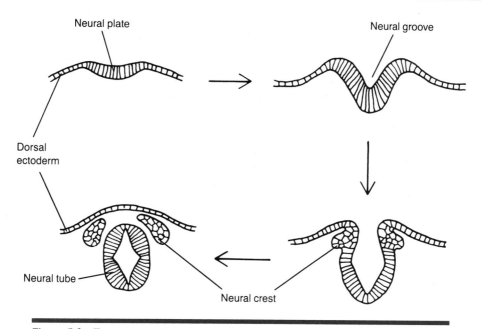

Figure 5-2 Transverse sections through the dorsal parts of a series of embryos to show how the neural plate gives rise to the neural tube and crests.

ventricular layer is the **mantle layer,** consisting of cells descended from those of the ventricular layer. The **marginal layer** is the outermost; it consists largely of neurites.

The cells in the mantle layer that become neurons are called **neuroblasts;** those that differentiate into neuroglial cells are **glioblasts.** In the spinal cord and brain stem, the marginal layer eventually comes to consist largely of masses of myelinated axons and their supporting glial cells, a tissue named **white matter,** from the color of the myelin. The mantle layer develops into masses of neuronal somata, dendrites, and synaptic connections. The color of such tissue in preserved anatomical specimens has given origin to the term **gray matter,** even though in the living state it is pink, owing to its rich blood supply. In the cerebrum, the cortex contains neurons derived from the mantle and marginal layers. The **ependyma** lining the ventricles and central canal is the remnant of the ventricular layer of the neural tube.

Spinal Cord, Brain Stem, and Cerebellum

The architecture of the neural tube remains recognizable in the adult spinal cord. The **alar plate,** consisting of the ventricular and mantle layers of the dorsal part of the tube, becomes the dorsal horn of the spinal gray matter. The **basal plate** in the ventral part of the tube becomes the ventral horn (Fig. 5-3). Neurons derived from the alar plate receive synapses from the primary sensory neurons in the spinal ganglia, whereas the neurons from the basal plate include the motor neurons that innervate striated skeletal muscle.

The alar and basal plates give rise to equivalent sets of neurons in the brain stem, even though this part of the neuraxis develops a shape quite different from that of the spinal cord (Fig. 5-3). The roof-plate of the medulla and pons is wide and thin. Consequently the alar plate lies laterally, and the basal plate lies medially, in the floor of the fourth ven-

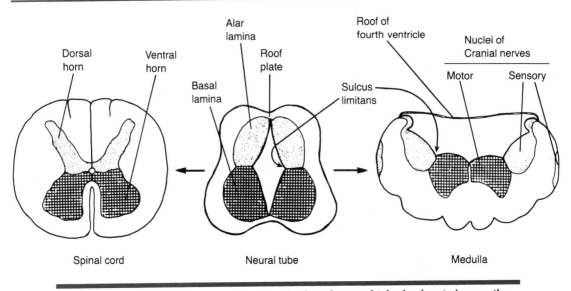

Figure 5-3 Diagrams of transverse sections showing how the neural tube develops to become the spinal cord (*Left*) and the brain stem (*Right*).

tricle. The **sulcus limitans,** separating the alar from the basal plate, persists in the floor of the fourth ventricle. Groups of motor and autonomic neurons lie medial to the sulcus limitans; groups of neurons lateral to the sulcus receive the incoming axons from the sensory ganglia of cranial nerves. The midbrain retains a tubular form, with most of the white matter in its ventral and lateral parts, and gray matter dorsal and ventral to the aqueduct.

The cerebellum arises as an outgrowth from the dorsolateral aspects of the brain stem. It has deep gray matter, associated with the rostal part of the roof of the fourth ventricle. and a cortex of gray matter on the external surface.

Diencephalon and Telencephalon

The rostral part of the neural tube grows much more than the parts that give rise to the brain stem and spinal cord, and flexures develop so that the brain comes to fill the cranium. The result is the formation of the cerebral hemispheres (Fig. 5-4). The arrangement of central gray matter and external white matter is conserved in the cerebral hemispheres, but not in an obvious way. The gray masses of the thalamus and hypothalamus flank the third ventricle, and external to them is the internal capsule, a band of white matter of great functional importance. The lateral ventricles have large gray masses, the corpora striata in their walls, with the white matter of the medullary centers of the hemispheres further out. The development of the cerebral hemispheres is complicated, however, by the formation of the cerebral cortex. This is formed from neuroblasts that migrate from the ventricular layer to the outside surface of the developing brain. As a result, most of the outside surface of the adult hemispheres consists of the gray matter of the cerebral cortex. The corpus callosum, a large mass of axons interconnecting the cortices of the two hemispheres, forms the roofs of both lateral ventricles.

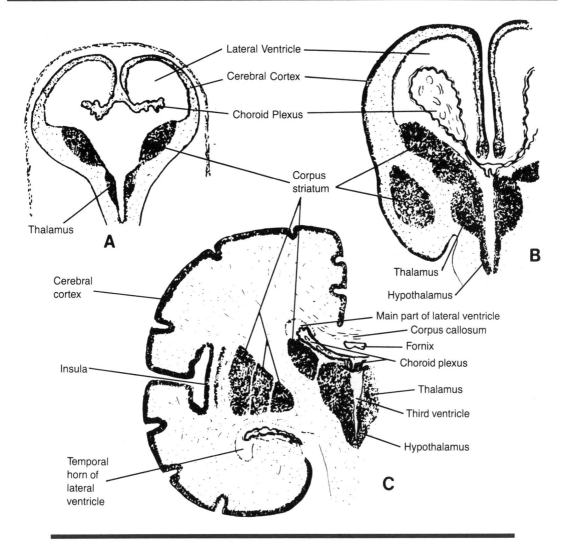

Figure 5-4 Stages in the development of the cerebral hemispheres. (**A**) 7 weeks after fertilization. (**B**) 17 weeks after fertilization. (**C**) The adult condition. (The anatomy of the cerebral hemisphere is described and illustrated in Chap. 11.) (Reproduced with permission from FitzGerald MJT: Human Embryology: A Regional Approach. Hagerstown, Harper & Row, 1978)

Formation of the Peripheral Nervous System

Some neural crest cells form aggregates close to the neural tube and become the spinal ganglia. Other groups of neural crest cells migrate ventrally to form the ganglia of the autonomic nervous system and the sensory ganglia of cranial nerves. The enteric nervous system is derived largely from the neural crest cells that also form the vagus nerve.

The cells giving rise to ganglia differentiate into both neurons and neuroglial cells. Other cells from the neural crest travel further to form the neuroglia (Schwann cells or neurolemmocytes) of all the peripheral nerves. The contribution of placodes to the peripheral nervous system has already been mentioned.

The most notable activity of neural crest cells is their migration, which has been intensively studied in recent years by making chick–quail chimeras. This is done by replacing a small piece of a chick embryo with a corresponding bit of tissue from a quail embryo. Development is then allowed to continue. The quail cells are incorporated into the growing chick, but can be recognized by virtue of a conspicuous lump of DNA in the interphase nucleus. This is absent from chick cells. It is reasonable to extrapolate to mammals from the results of experiments with chick–quail chimeras, because the conclusions correspond closely to those derived from "static" observations made on graded series of embryos of different ages. The anatomical organization of the peripheral nervous system is, in any case, similar in all vertebrates.

Special Sense Organs

The organs of smell, sight, taste, hearing, and equilibration are all derived, at least in part, from ectodermal placodes rather than from the neuroectoderm.

The **olfactory placode,** which is part of the larger nasal placode, forms the olfactory epithelium. This consists of neurons and supporting cells that are always in contact with the external environment. The axons of the olfactory neurons grow towards and enter the most rostral part of the embryonic forebrain. Even in adult mammals, the neurons of the olfactory epithelium can be replaced from a population of undifferentiated precursor cells (see Chap. 14).

The development of the **eye** (Fig. 5-5) is a process of great complexity. Initially an outgrowth from the diencephalon forms the optic stalk, dilated at its end to form an optic vesicle. Invagination of the vesicle forms a two-layered optic cup, which will become the retina. When the optic vesicle touches the ectoderm on the surface, a placode is formed and it sinks in towards the developing neural components of the eye. It will become the lens. Mesodermal cells, attracted into the fissure between the developing optic cup and the lens placode, eventually form the choroid, iris, sclera, vitreous body, and blood vessels. The eye is largely formed by the end of the 7th week after conception.

Taste cells are derived from the ordinary ectoderm of the mouth. They acquire their chemical sensitivity when they are contacted by the growing axons of neurons in the sensory ganglia of the VIIth, IXth or Xth cranial nerves (see Chap. 20). Small groups of the innervated cells constitute **taste buds.** Most of them are on the tongue.

The **otic placode** appears 3 weeks after conception; it sinks into the mesoderm and forms the otic vesicle, which will become the sensory epithelia of both the cochlea (for hearing) and the vestibular labyrinth (for equilibration), as well as the sensory ganglia of the cranial nerve (VIII) that serves the sensory cells. The neuroglia of the vestibulocochlear nerve originates from the cranial neural crest. The middle ear is an endodermal derivative, being an outgrowth of the pharynx. The ossicles are mesodermal. The external ear is a late development, the external meatus opens in the 6th month of intrauterine life, and the growth of the pinna continues for years after birth.

Developmental Abnormalities of the Central Nervous System

The most serious abnormalities to arise during development of the nervous system are due to failure of closure of the neural groove. Nervous tissue is exposed on the dorsal surface

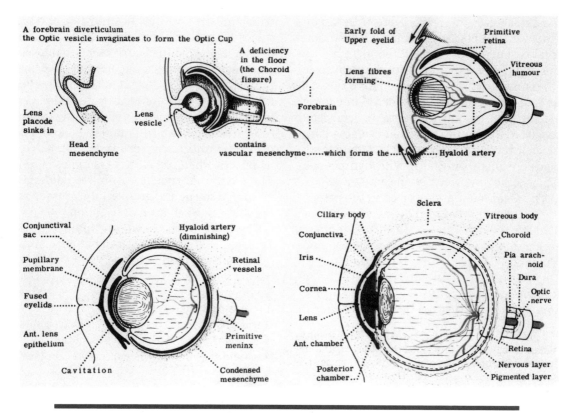

Figure 5-5 Stages in the development of the eye. (The anatomy of the eye is discussed and illustrated in Chap. 18.) (Reproduced with permission from Wendell Smith CP, Williams PL, Treadgold S: Basic Human Embryology, 3rd ed. London, Pitman Publishing, 1984).

of the body, because there is also failure of development of the overlying meninges, vertebral arches, and skin. If the neural groove does not close at its cranial end, the whole forebrain and the overlying skull and scalp will be missing, although the face and eyes will be formed. This condition is called **anencephaly** (meaning "no brain"), and the afflicted individual is either stillborn or survives for only a few hours. The corresponding condition at the caudal end of the central nervous system is **myeloschisis** ("split spinal cord"), with extensive exposure of nonfunctional nervous tissue in the lumbosacral region. Myeloschisis and anencephaly often occur together.

Myeloschisis is the most severe form of **spina bifida,** a condition in which there are missing vertebral arches, nearly always in the lumbar region. In the less severe varieties, the spinal cord and its immediate coverings (the leptomeninges) are formed and there is a covering of skin, but the associated mesodermal structures are defective. Thus there may be a **meningomyelocele,** with the spinal cord protruding as a swelling through the hole formed by the missing vertebral arches and dura. (The dura is the strong collagenous membrane that lines the cranium and spinal canal.) If the spinal cord remains near the vertebral bodies, there is a cystic swelling composed of leptomeningeal tissue and cerebrospinal fluid. This is a **meningocele.** The least severe of these conditions is **spina bifida occulta,** in which the dura is intact but one or more vertebral arches are missing. Spina bifida occulta may cause no symptoms, or it may be blamed for otherwise undiagnosed pain in the back. Meningomyelocele and meningocele can be corrected surgically, but often the child remains paraplegic (lower limbs paralyzed). Meningomyelocele is often associated with hydrocephalus, a condition discussed in Chapter 30.

The abnormalities described in the preceding two paragraphs are anatomically obvious. Though they are among the most common serious disorders of development, they are not common diseases. Mental retardation is a common disorder. Usually the cause is unknown, but in some cases there is a chromosomal abnormality, as in **Down's syndrome,*** in

---

* JLH Down (1828–1896) was the English physician who, in 1866, described the physical and behavioral features of the disease now known as "trisomy-21," "mongolism," or "Down's syndrome."

which all the somatic cells have 47 chromosomes instead of the normal 46. Factors inducing abnormalities are called **teratogens.** Many have been suggested, but few have been proved to result in human disease. The best known teratogens are certain diseases, notably syphilis and rubella, thalidomide (an obsolete sedative), ionizing radiation, and most cytotoxic (anticancer) drugs. A teratogen has its effects when the embryo is exposed to it. Thus maternal rubella can induce defective closure of the neural groove only between the 3rd and 4th week after conception.

The brain of the newborn infant is easily damaged by injury, endocrine abnormalities (especially hypothyroidism), and metabolic insults such as malnutrition. When suitable treatment is available, as it is for several endocrine and metabolic disorders, it must be started as soon as possible. When treatment is delayed beyond the 3rd postnatal month, the mental deficiency is usually no longer reversible.

Chapter 6

Anatomy of the Peripheral Nervous System

Spinal and Cranial Nerves

The most conspicuous superficial feature of the spinal cord is the abundance of **rootlets** of spinal nerves. On each side the rootlets form two continuous lines, one in a dorsolateral position and one in a ventrolateral position. Groups of rootlets join together to form dorsal and ventral **roots.** Each dorsal root bears a ganglion; ventral roots do not have ganglia. At each segmental level the dorsal and ventral roots fuse to make a mixed **spinal nerve,** which is also often called a "root." This leaves the spinal canal by way of an intervertebral foramen. The letters **C, T, L,** and **S** denote the cervical, thoracic, lumbar, and sacral levels. Thus the sixth cervical nerve is commonly called "C6." Nerves C1 to C7 pass through foramina *above* the corresponding vertebrae; nerve C8 leaves the spinal canal between the arches of vertebrae C7 and T1. The 12 thoracic nerves and 5 lumbar nerves pass *below* the corresponding vertebrae. The sacral vertebrae are fused, and the pairs of nerves S1 to S5 emerge through foramina in the sacrum. The single pair of coccygeal nerves emerges from the caudal end of the canal of the sacrum.

The commonest disease affecting spinal nerves is compression by a protrusion derived from an intervertebral disc. In the cervical spine, this affects the root corresponding to the vertebral level (commonly C5, 6, or 7), but in the lumbar spine a protrusion from a disc presses on a nerve one or two segments rostral to its exit foramen. For example, a protrusion from the L4-L5 disc commonly compresses nerve S1.

Symptoms of compression of a spinal root include abnormal sensation in the region supplied with sensory fibers and weakness of the muscles supplied by the nerve. Chapter 7 contains information used for clinical recognition of segmental levels.

The 12 **cranial nerves** connect the brain with peripheral structures. The nerves are numbered and named as follows: I—olfactory; II—optic (not really a nerve, but part of the central nervous system); III—oculomotor; IV—trochlear; V—trigeminal; VI—abducent; VII—facial; VIII—vestibulocochlear; IX—glossopharyngeal; X—vagus; XI—accessory; XII—hypoglossal.

Somatic and Visceral Innervation

There are two divisions of the peripheral nervous system that overlap to some extent. The **somatic** division is concerned with sensation arising in skin, muscles, and joints and with the motor innervation of skeletal striated muscle. The **visceral** division is concerned with internal organs and with blood vessels and glands everywhere. The special senses are considered to be visceral when concerned with feeding (smell, taste), but are otherwise classified as somatic.

Somatic Nervous System

The sensory neurons have their somata in **dorsal root ganglia,** which are swellings on the dorsal roots of the spinal nerves. These ganglia are simply cell-stations and do not contain synapses. Equivalent ganglia occur on some of the cranial nerves. The sensory neurons are unipolar (see Chap. 2, Fig. 2-2). The single neurite of such a neuron is called an axon; its long peripheral branch goes to a sensory receptor, and its short central branch enters the spinal cord or brain stem.

The somata of **motor neurons** lie in the ventral horn of the grey matter of the spinal cord or in appropriate cranial nerve nuclei in the brain stem. The axons of spinal motor neurons leave the cord in the ventral roots of the segmental nerves. The ventral root joins the dorsal root (Fig. 6-1), and the motor axons are eventually distributed to muscles. Each axon branches within the muscle to supply several muscle fibers. "Several" may mean hundreds in the bulky muscles of the thigh, or fewer than 10 in muscles responsible for delicate movements, as in the hand or the extraocular muscles. The motor neuron, its axon, and all the muscle fibers it supplies constitute a **motor unit.** An impulse conducted along the axon of a motor neuron causes all the muscle fibers of the motor unit to contract simultaneously.

The dorsal and ventral roots join near the intervertebral foramen. The mixed spinal nerve, which is also called a "root," divides into dorsal and ventral **primary rami** (a "ramus" is a branch). The dorsal primary ramus

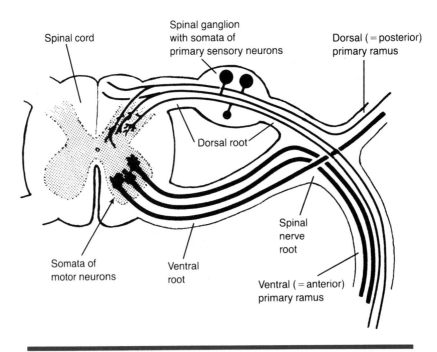

Figure 6-1 Formation of a spinal nerve from the dorsal and ventral roots. Neurons concerned with visceral innervation are not included in this diagram, but are illustrated in Chapter 27 (Fig. 27-1).

supplies the skin of the dorsal surface of the trunk and those muscles that are intimately associated with the vertebral column. The ventral primary ramus is larger and supplies the limbs and the ventral parts of the trunk. A single nerve supplying a muscle or an area of skin in a limb contains axons from more than one spinal nerve. The mixing of axons from nearby roots occur in **plexuses**—the brachial plexus for the upper limb and the lumbosacral plexus for the lower limb (Fig. 6-2). In a plexus, nerves join, separate, and rejoin, and the exchange of axons produces muscular

and cutaneous nerves with mixed segmental origins. In the skin, a further redistribution of axons peripherally results in the formation of distinct though overlapping areas (dermatomes; see Chap. 7) supplied by individual dorsal roots.

Visceral Nervous System

Skeletal muscle fibers are innervated by neurons of the central nervous system. Smooth muscle, cardiac muscle, and glands, on the

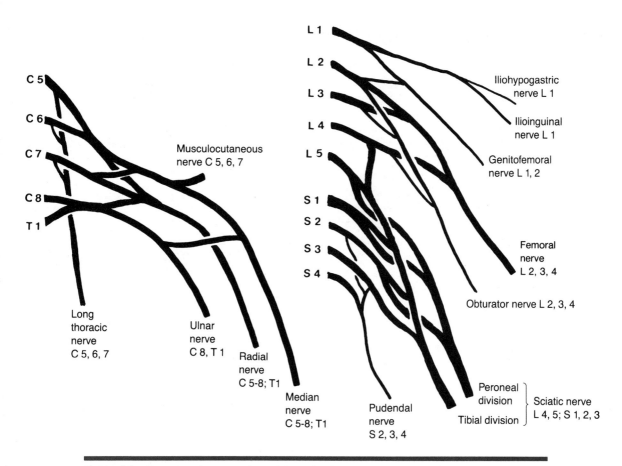

Figure 6-2 Examples of plexuses formed from segmental nerves in man. The **brachial plexus** (*Left*) is for the innervation of the upper limb. Most of the nerves from the **lumbosacral plexus** (*Right*) supply the lower limb. The diagrams of both plexuses have been simplified by omitting some small nerves.

other hand, are supplied by the axons of neurons whose somata lie peripherally, in ganglia. These ganglia, with the nerves entering and leaving them, constitute the **autonomic nervous system.** *Unlike a sensory ganglion, an autonomic ganglion contains synapses.* The thin myelinated (Group B) axons of neurons in the spinal cord or brain stem are the **preganglionic fibers,** which contact the neurons in the ganglion. **Postganglionic fibers** are the unmyelinated (Group C) axons of the cells of the ganglion. They are distributed to the organs receiving autonomic innervation.

Preganglionic autonomic axons leave the brain stem in some of the cranial nerves (III, VII, IX, X) and in the ventral roots of some of the spinal nerves (T1-L3; S2-S4). One conspicuous set of autonomic ganglia is associated with the spinal nerves and with the branches of the abdominal aorta. These ganglia and their afferent and efferent nerves constitute the **sympathetic** division of the autonomic nervous system. Other ganglia, in the head, thorax, abdomen, and pelvis, lie close to the organs they supply and belong to the **parasympathetic** division. The third division of the autonomic system is the **enteric nervous system,** contained in the wall of the alimentary canal from esophagus to rectum. The anatomy and functions of the autonomic nervous system are described in more detail in Chapter 27.

The **sensory neurons** that supply the viscera have their cell-bodies in dorsal root and cranial nerve ganglia, together with somatic sensory neurons. The distal branches of the visceral sensory axons pass through the appropriate autonomic ganglia (without making any synaptic contacts there) and are distributed in the same nerves as the efferent autonomic fibers. Visceral afferent signals concerned with physiological regulation do not give rise to consciously experienced sensations. Pain from diseased internal organs is commonly "referred" to parts of the body that receive somatic innervation from the same segmental nerves.

Nerve Components

Every peripheral nerve contains populations of axons with different functions. Each type of axonal population is a **nerve component.** Nerve components mentioned in this chapter are: somatic efferent (motor), visceral efferent (pre- and postganglionic autonomic) and somatic and visceral afferent. An appreciation of components is helpful in understanding the cranial nerves (see Chap. 20).

Nerve Endings

The microscopic structure and the functions of sensory and motor nerve endings are considered in Chapter 13.

Chapter 7

The Spinal Cord

The adult human spinal cord extends about 45 cm from the foramen magnum in the base of the skull to the lower border of the first lumbar vertebral body. The cord is 1 to 1.5 cm across, being narrowest in the thoracic region and widest in the lower cervical and lumbosacral regions. A central core of gray matter is surrounded by white matter.

The spinal cord is shorter than the spinal canal, so a needle may be inserted between the arches of vertebrae below L2 without risk of injuring the spinal cord. This procedure, known as **lumbar puncture** or spinal tap, is used to obtain specimens of cerebrospinal fluid (see Chap. 30). The nerve roots in the spinal canal are harmlessly pushed aside by the needle.

Segmentation

Early in embryonic development, segments (neuromeres) of the neural tube become imperceptibly fused. In the adult, segmentation is evident only in the spinal nerves and the structures they supply. The areas of skin whose dermis is derived from the somites of the embryo are known as **dermatomes.** Groups of muscles are derived from the myotomes, but are not given this name in the mature condition.

Dermatomes

Each dermatome is supplied with sensory nerve fibers from an individual dorsal root.

On the trunk, the dermatomes form a pattern of bands. The segmental pattern in the limbs is less obvious (Fig. 7-1). Adjacent dermatomes overlap by approximately the width of one dermatome. Thus any point on the skin receives sensory innervation from three segmental nerves, though the middle one provides more fibers than those above and below. The overlap is greater for gentle touch than for painful stimuli.

Certain dermatomes are worth remembering for clinical purposes. The important landmarks are the following:

(C1—usually has no dorsal root)
C2—occipital region of head
C5—tip of shoulder
C6—thumb
C8—little finger
T4—T5—nipple
T10—umbilicus
L3—front of knee
L5—big toe
S1—little toe; heel
S3 and below—genitalia; anal area

Groups of Muscles

Muscles are supplied by nerves of mixed segmental origin from the limb plexuses. The nerve to a muscle contains the motor fibers that cause contraction and the sensory fibers that supply the muscle spindles and the nerve endings in tendons. Branches of the nerves to

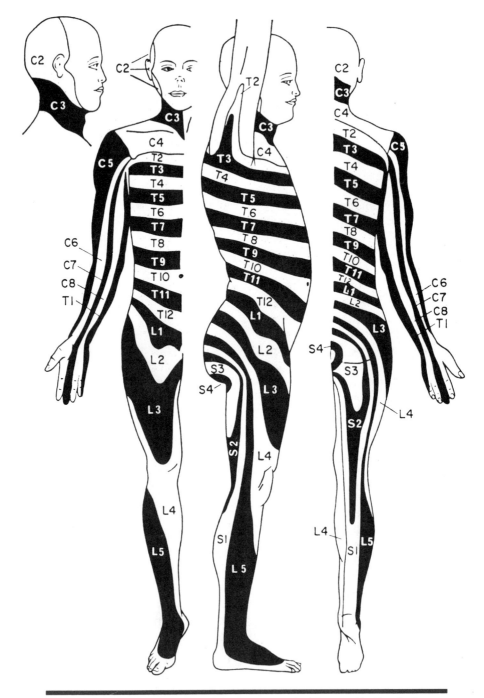

Figure 7-1   The segmental innervation (**dermatomes**) of human skin. For the face, see Chapter 20 (Fig. 20-1). (Reproduced with permission from Walton, Sir J: Essentials of Neurology, 5th ed. London, Pitman Publishing, 1982)

muscles also go to sensory endings in and around the joints moved by the muscles. Segmental organization of muscular innervation is not as clearly defined as that of the skin. Spinal roots control groups of muscles that cooperate to make movements.

Some important examples are the following:

C5–C6—flexion of elbow ("biceps jerk")
C7–C8—extension of elbow ("triceps jerk")
C8–T1—small muscles of hand
L2–L3—quadriceps ("knee jerk")
S1–S2—calf muscles ("ankle jerk")

The "jerk" reflexes mentioned in parentheses are elicited by suddenly stretching the muscles by tapping the tendon with a rubber-covered hammer. The monosynaptic stretch reflex causes a contraction that is observed visually. The tendon-jerk reflexes test both the sensory and the motor innervation of muscles. It is also necessary to evaluate strength directly.

Levels of the Spinal Cord

Recognition of the segmental level of a transverse section of the spinal cord is not a test of parrot-like memory, but an exercise in common sense. The volume of gray matter is greatest at the levels concerned with the limbs, which are rich in skin and muscle. At levels T1 to L3, neurons are also present for the innervation of the sympathetic ganglia. These cells occupy a small "lateral horn" in their segments. Equivalent cells for the sacral parasympathetic system (S2–S4) do not influence the cross-sectional shape of the gray matter. The numbers of fibers in both the ascending and descending tracts of the white matter are greatest rostrally, and least caudally. Thus the cross-sectional area of the white matter is greatest in the cervical, and smallest in the sacral, segments.

Figure 7-2 illustrates selected levels of the spinal cord. The student should note the application of the principles outlined in the preceding paragraph.

Anatomy and Circuitry of the Spinal Gray Matter

The spinal gray matter is subdivided into longitudinal columns of neurons, the **laminae of Rexed,** named after the Swedish neuroanatomist who first described them in 1952.

The laminae (Fig. 7-3) are numbered from I to X, from the tip of the dorsal horn to the area around the central canal. Lamina VI is present only in the segments that supply limbs. Lamina IX is not a true lamina, but a set of columns of motor neurons; these columns are embedded in laminae VII and VIII. Lamina VII is a large area between the dorsal and ventral horns, also known as the intermediate gray matter. In the middle segments

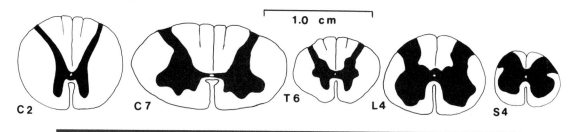

Figure 7-2 Transverse sections of the human spinal cord at various levels.

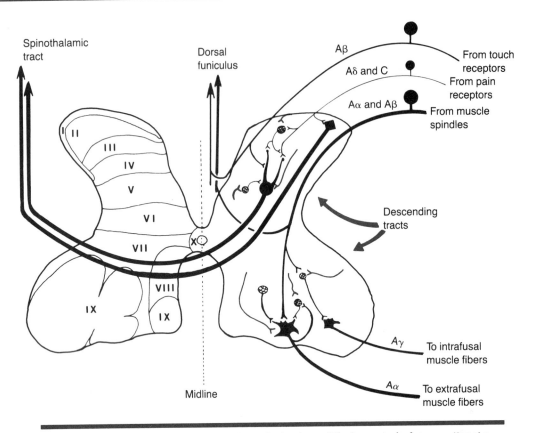

Figure 7-3   The *left* half of this diagram shows the laminae of the human spinal gray matter at a lumbar level. The *right* side shows some of the principal cells and interneurons and their connections.

of the spinal cord, lamina VII contains two prominent columns of cells. The **thoracic nucleus** (also called *nucleus dorsalis* or Clarke's column, after Jacob Clarke (1817–1880), the English anatomist who described it) is present at the root of the dorsal horn in segments C8 to L3. It contains the neuronal somata that give rise to the axons constituting the dorsal spinocerebellar tract. The lateral horn, in segments T1 to L3, is also called the **intermediolateral cell column.** It contains the cell-bodies of the preganglionic sympathetic fibers. This cell column is also present in segments S2–S4,

for the preganglionic sacral parasympathetic nerves.

The columns of neurons constituting lamina IX contain principal cells and interneurons. The former are **motor neurons** whose myelinated axons leave the spinal cord in the ventral roots and supply skeletal muscle fibers. The largest motor neurons have the longest axons. Small motor neurons are those with short axons and those that supply the intrafusal fibers of muscle spindles (see Chap. 13). The medially located components of lamina IX supply axial muscles, whereas motor

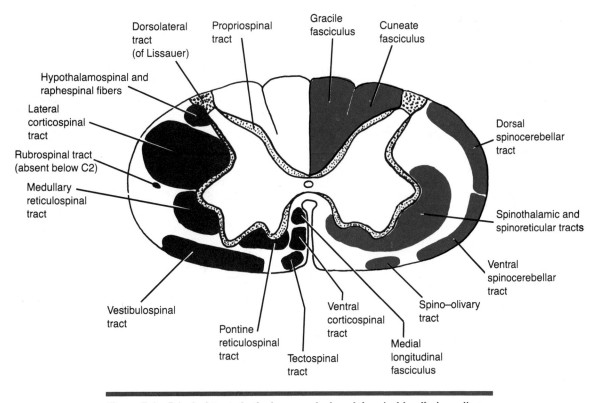

Figure 7-4 Principal tracts in the human spinal cord (cervical level). Ascending fibers are colored; descending fibers are black.

neurons for the limbs are more laterally placed. Two special columns of motor neurons are present in the ventral horns of the cervical cord. These are the **accessory nucleus** (C1–C5), which gives rise to the spinal root of cranial nerve XI, and the **phrenic nucleus** (C3–C5), whose neurons supply the diaphragm through the phrenic nerve.

Primary afferent axons entering from the dorsal roots terminate in all the laminae of the dorsal horn. Ascending tracts concerned with sensation (the spinothalamic and spinoreticular tracts) consist largely of the axons of cells in laminae I and V. Descending tracts from the brain are concerned with movement and with the modulation of the upward trans-

mission of sensory information. Descending fibers therefore terminate in all the laminae. Those involved in movement end mainly in lamina VII, though some end in laminae VIII and IX. Descending fibers that influence the spinothalamic and spinoreticular tracts end principally in the dorsal horn. These and some other neuronal connections are shown in Figure 7-3.

Tracts of the Spinal White Matter

The positions of the more important tracts are shown in Figure 7-4. The level chosen for this illustration is cervical, because all the tracts

Table 7-1. Tracts of the Spinal Cord

Name of Tract (For position in cord, see Fig. 7-4)	Origin	Termination (Roman numerals refer to Rexed's laminae)	Function
Propriospinal fibers	Spinal gray (V–VIII)	Spinal gray at other levels	Reflexes within spinal cord
Dorsolateral tract (of Lissauer*)	Dorsal root ganglion	Spinal gray above and below level of root (I–V)	Pain and temperature sensation (Chap. 15)
Dorsal funiculus (consists of cuneate and gracile fasciculi)	Ipsilateral dorsal root ganglion	**Cuneate fasciculus:** Ipsilateral cuneate nucleus	Discriminative tactile sensation and conscious proprioception, from upper limb (Chap. 15)
		Ipsilateral accessory cuneate nucleus	Unconscious proprioception (Chap. 24)
		Gracile fasciculus: Ipsilateral gracile nucleus	Discriminative tactile sensation, lower limb (Chap. 15)
		Ipsilateral thoracic nucleus (VII)	Conscious *and* unconscious proprioception, lower limb (Chap. 15, 24)
Spinothalamic tract	Contralateral dorsal horn (mainly I & V); fibers cross near central canal before ascending	Thalamus (VPL and some other nuclei)	Pain, temperature and touch (Chap. 15)
Spinoreticular tracts	Spinal gray of both sides (V–VII)	Medullary and pontine reticular formation, of both sides	Consciousness and arousal (Chap. 21) General awareness of pain (Chap. 15)
Dorsal spinocerebellar tract	Ipsilateral thoracic nucleus	Ipsilateral cortex of spinocerebellum	Unconscious proprioceptive control of movement of lower limb (Chap. 24)
		Branches to ipsilateral nucleus Z in medulla	Conscious proprioception, lower limb (Chap. 15)
Ventral spinocerebellar tract	Spinal gray (largely contralateral)	Cortex of spinocerebellum (after a second decussation within the cerebellum)	Unconscious proprioceptive control of movement (Chaps. 9, 24)

(Continued)

Table 7-1. Tracts of the Spinal Cord *(Continued)*

Name of Tract (For position in cord, see Fig. 7-4)	Origin	Termination (Roman numerals refer to Rexed's laminae)	Function
Lateral corticospinal tract (pyramidal tract)	Contralateral cerebral cortex (frontal and parietal lobes)	Dorsal and ventral horns of spinal gray (mainly IV–IX)	Modulates activity in sensory tracts (Chap. 15) Control of skilled movements (Chaps. 23, 24)
Ventral corticospinal tract	As for above tract, but ipsilateral	Fibers cross at segmental levels and then go to same sites as lateral tract	Same as for lateral corticospinal tract
Vestibulospinal tract ("lateral vestibulospinal tract")	Ipsilateral lateral vestibular nucleus	Ipsilateral ventral horn (VII, VIII)	Control of muscles that maintain upright posture (Chaps. 17, 24)
Medial longitudinal fasciculus (descending component[†])	Ipsilateral medial vestibular nucleus	Ipsilateral ventral horn, upper cervical segments of spinal cord	Position of head (Chaps. 17, 19)
Reticulospinal tracts	Medullary and pontine reticular formation, bilaterally	Spinal gray (VII–IX), bilaterally	Control of movement (Chaps. 23, 24)
Tectospinal tract	Contralateral superior colliculus	Ventral horn of upper cervical spinal cord	Position of head, in association with eye movements
Raphespinal tract	Raphe nuclei of medulla	Dorsal horn (I–III)	Suppresses pain (Chaps. 15, 21)
Hypothalamospinal tract	Hypothalamus	Segments T1–L1 and S2–S4 (VII)	Control of autonomic nervous system (Chaps. 26, 27)
Solitariospinal tract	Solitary nucleus	Probably same as hypothalamospinal fibers	Probably control of autonomic nervous system

[*] H. Lissauer (1861–1891) was a German neurologist.
[†] This tract is sometimes called the "medial vestibulospinal tract."

are largest in the rostral part of the cord. It should be noted that the positions of some tracts are not precisely known in man, and adjacent tracts certainly overlap. Table 7-1 is provided for reference. It summarizes the origins, terminations, and functions of the major spinal tracts and refers the reader to other chapters where the functions are discussed.

Spinal Reflexes

An important function of the descending tracts is to modify simple reflexes within the spinal cord. The reflexes alone can regulate only very simple movements. Appropriately facilitated or inhibited by the brain, the reflex movements are made purposeful. (Circuitry involved in the control of movement is reviewed in Chapters 23 and 24.) Three important spinal reflexes must now be described.

The **stretch reflex** is monosynaptic. The neuromuscular spindles initiate impulses in sensory axons when a muscle is stretched. Intraspinal branches of the sensory axons are presynaptic and excitatory to motor neurons that supply the same muscle. The simplest form of the stretch reflex is seen in the "tendon jerks"—any muscle will contract if its tendon is suddenly pulled. Spindles are also stretched when their own (intrafusal) muscle fibers, supplied by gamma motor neurons, contract. Excitation of the sensory endings then stimulates the alpha motor neurons and causes contraction of the ordinary (extrafusal) fibers of the muscle. Both the alpha and

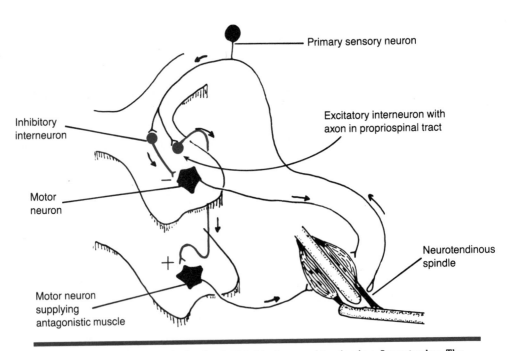

Figure 7-5 Pathway for a spinal reflex initiated by increased tension in a flexor tendon. The reflex causes relaxation of the flexor and contraction of the extensor muscle.

the gamma motor neurons are influenced by descending tracts.

Neurotendinous spindles detect the tension in a tendon. They initiate polysynaptic reflexes that inhibit the motor neurons and, through neurons with axons in the propriospinal tract, excite the neurons that innervate antagonistic muscles. These reflexes are important for smooth movements, for the stability of joints, and for protecting muscles and tendons against injuriously strong contraction.

The **flexor reflex** is also polysynaptic. It is a defensive response to a painful stimulus felt at the end of a limb. The flexor muscles of the limb contract, the extensors are inhibited, and with a strong stimulus there is extension of the contralateral limb.

Figure 7-5 illustrates a reflex involving tendon receptors. Using the information presented in the preceding paragraphs, the student should be able to make similar diagrams of the other spinal reflexes.

Chapter 8

The Brain Stem

The brain stem consists of the mesencephalon (**midbrain**) and rhombencephalon (**hindbrain**), excluding the cerebellum. The rhombencephalic parts of the brain stem are the **pons** and the **medulla oblongata.** The brain stem contains the nuclei of most of the cranial nerves, several other important nuclei, and various ascending and descending tracts of fibers. The midbrain is connected with the diencephalon and the telencephalon rostrally. Caudally, the medulla is continuous with the spinal cord. Laterally and dorsally, the cerebellum is connected to the brain stem by three cerebellar peduncles on each side. The central cavity of the midbrain is the **cerebral aqueduct.** This continues rostrally into the third ventricle (in the diencephalon), and caudally into the **fourth ventricle** (in the pons and upper medulla). The fourth ventricle is narrowed caudally, to become the **central canal** of the lower part of the medulla and of the spinal cord.

Surface Features of the Medulla, Pons, and Midbrain

The major landmarks of the ventral and lateral surfaces of the brain stem, including the roots of the cranial nerves, are shown in Figure 8-1. The components, functions and central connections of the cranial nerves are discussed in other chapters. The following are the other important landmarks:

Basis Pedunculi. (See Figs. 8-7, 8-8.) This consists of the axons of neurons in the cerebral cortex. They are continuing caudally from the internal capsule of the cerebral hemisphere, and they will end in the pontine nuclei (Fig. 8-5, 8-6), the medulla, and the spinal cord.

Basilar Part of Pons. Contains the left and right groups of pontine nuclei and their axons, which cross the midline and go to the cerebellum as the middle cerebellar peduncle. Descending fibers from the cerebral cortex traverse this part of the pons in small bundles.

Pyramid. This consists of corticospinal fibers which, having emerged from the basilar part of the pons, form a compact and prominent tract on the ventral surface of the medulla. At the caudal end of the medulla, most of the corticospinal fibers cross the midline in the decussation of the pyramids.

Olive. This eminence is raised by the inferior olivary nucleus (Fig. 8-4), an important source of fibers going to the cerebellum.

Cerebellar peduncles. The superior cerebellar peduncle joins the cerebellum to the midbrain; the middle peduncle, which is the largest, consists of pontocerebellar fibers; the inferior cerebellar peduncle connects the medulla with the cerebellum.

Roof of the Fourth Ventricle. The roof of the fourth ventricle consists of the superior medullary velum (a thin layer of white

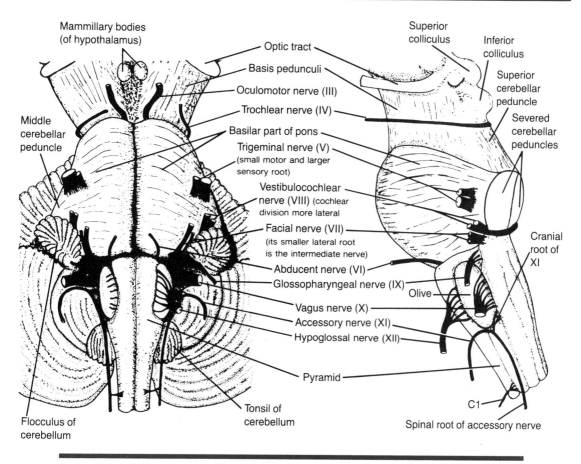

Figure 8-1 Principal features of the ventral (*Left*) and lateral (*Right*) aspects of the human brain stem. In the right-hand figure, the cerebellum has been removed by cutting through its peduncles.

matter bridging the inverted V formed by the two superior cerebellar peduncles), part of the cerebellum, and the inferior medullary velum (a thin membrane made of ependyma and connective tissue bridging the V formed by the inferior peduncles). Other features of the roof of the fourth ventricle are discussed in Chapter 30, in connection with the circulation of the cerebrospinal fluid.

If the three cerebellar peduncles of each side are transected, the cerebellum is easily

removed, revealing the dorsal surface of the brain stem. This consists of the tectum of the midbrain, the floor of the fourth ventricle, and the dorsal surface of the closed part of the medulla (Fig. 8-2). The following are the major landmarks:

Superior colliculus. This receives some of the axons of the optic tract and is mainly concerned with eye movements.

Inferior colliculus. A nucleus in the auditory pathway. The four colliculi (a word from

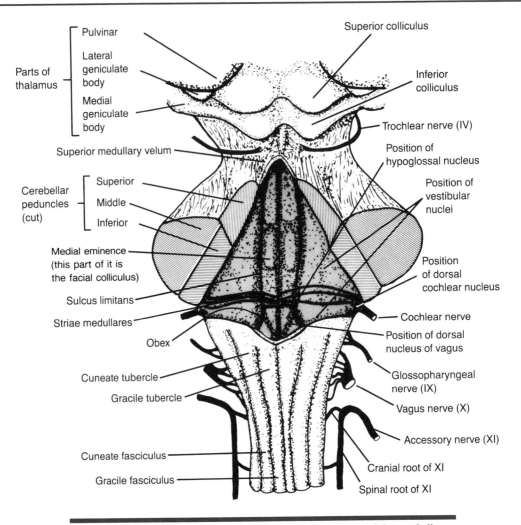

Parts of thalamus
- Pulvinar
- Lateral geniculate body
- Medial geniculate body

Superior medullary velum

Cerebellar peduncles (cut)
- Superior
- Middle
- Inferior

Medial eminence (this part of it is the facial colliculus)

Sulcus limitans

Striae medullares

Obex

Cuneate tubercle

Gracile tubercle

Cuneate fasciculus

Gracile fasciculus

Superior colliculus

Inferior colliculus

Trochlear nerve (IV)

Position of hypoglossal nucleus

Position of vestibular nuclei

Position of dorsal cochlear nucleus

Cochlear nerve

Position of dorsal nucleus of vagus

Glossopharyngeal nerve (IX)

Vagus nerve (X)

Accessory nerve (XI)

Cranial root of XI

Spinal root of XI

Figure 8-2   Dorsal view of the human brain stem after removal of the cerebellum to expose the floor of the fourth ventricle. (For other features of the ventricle, including its roof, see Fig. 30-2 in Chap. 30.)

the Latin, meaning "little hills") constitute the **tectum** (which means "roof").

Sulcus limitans. This groove separates the medial part of the floor of the fourth ventricle from the lateral part. The area medial to the sulcus limitans corresponds to the ventral horn of the spinal gray matter, whereas

the area lateral to the sulcus corresponds to the dorsal horn.

The **vagal trigone, hypoglossal trigone,** and **vestibular area** indicate underlying nuclei of cranial nerves X, XII, and VIII, respectively, in the medulla.

The **facial colliculus** is a poorly defined eminence raised by fibers from the motor nucleus of the facial nerve looping around the nucleus of the abducent nerve, in the caudal part of the pons.

The **striae medullares** are conspicuous, but perhaps not very important, bundles of axons going to the cerebellum.

The **obex** is the place where the fourth ventricle narrows caudally to become the central canal of the closed part of the medulla. Note that the "open" part is open only after

the roof of the fourth ventricle has been removed with the cerebellum.

The **lateral recess** of the diamond-shaped fourth ventricle extends over the upper end of the inferior cerebellar peduncle, where the roof is deficient. This lateral aperture is often occupied by a tuft of choroid plexus.

The **gracile** and **cuneate tubercles** indicate the gracile and cuneate nuclei, which are important nuclei in some of the somatic sensory pathways.

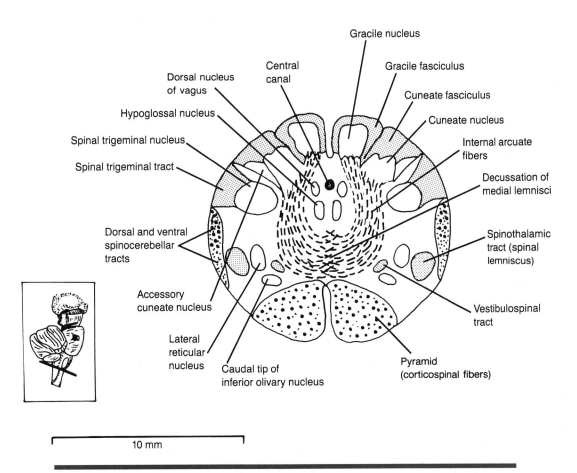

10 mm

Figure 8-3 Transverse section through the closed part of the medulla showing the major nuclei and tracts.

Internal Structure of the Brain Stem

Full comprehension of the anatomy of the brain stem can be obtained only after laborious study of a series of transverse sections in conjunction with pictures and a descriptive text. No attempt is made here to provide a detailed description. The positions of the largest and most important nuclei and tracts are shown at selected levels in Figures 8-3 to 8-8.

The spaces separating the major nuclei and tracts from one another, at all levels of the brain stem, contain the nuclei of the **reticular formation** (see Chap. 21). The term **tegmentum** identifies the dorsal part of the pons, together with those parts of the midbrain between the tectum and the substantia nigra.

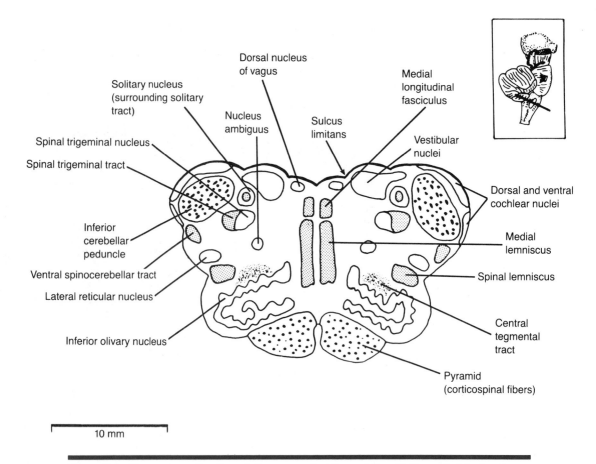

Figure 8-4   Transverse section through the open part of the medulla with the roof of the fourth ventricle removed.

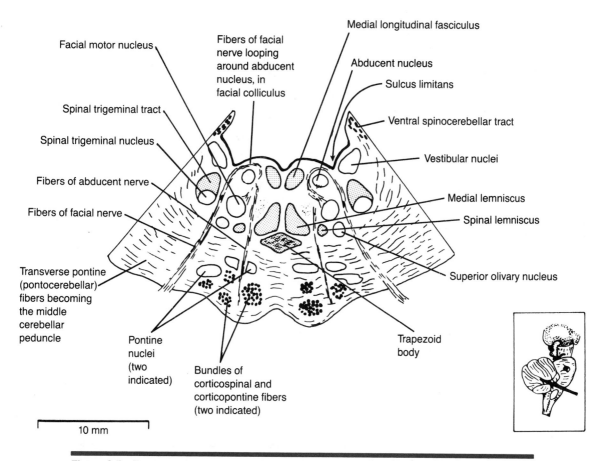

Facial motor nucleus

Fibers of facial nerve looping around abducent nucleus, in facial colliculus

Medial longitudinal fasciculus

Abducent nucleus

Spinal trigeminal tract

Sulcus limitans

Spinal trigeminal nucleus

Ventral spinocerebellar tract

Fibers of abducent nerve

Vestibular nuclei

Fibers of facial nerve

Medial lemniscus

Spinal lemniscus

Transverse pontine (pontocerebellar) fibers becoming the middle cerebellar peduncle

Superior olivary nucleus

Pontine nuclei (two indicated)

Bundles of corticospinal and corticopontine fibers (two indicated)

Trapezoid body

10 mm

Figure 8-5 Transverse section at the level (see inset) of the pontomedullary junction.

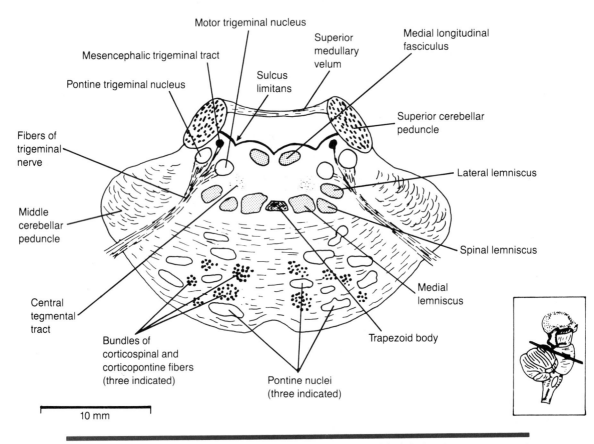

Figure 8-6   Transverse section through the pons at the level of the trigeminal nerve.

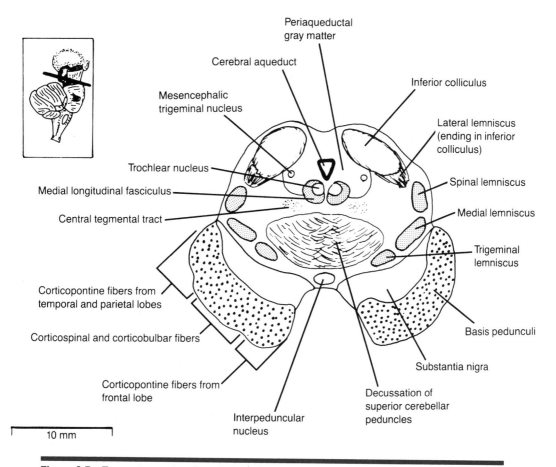

Periaqueductal
gray matter

Cerebral aqueduct

Inferior colliculus

Mesencephalic
trigeminal nucleus

Lateral lemniscus
(ending in inferior
colliculus)

Trochlear nucleus

Spinal lemniscus

Medial longitudinal fasciculus

Medial lemniscus

Central tegmental tract

Trigeminal
lemniscus

Corticopontine fibers from
temporal and parietal lobes

Basis pedunculi

Corticospinal and corticobulbar fibers

Substantia nigra

Corticopontine fibers from
frontal lobe

Decussation of
superior cerebellar
peduncles

Interpeduncular
nucleus

10 mm

Figure 8-7   Transverse section through the midbrain at the level of the inferior colliculus.

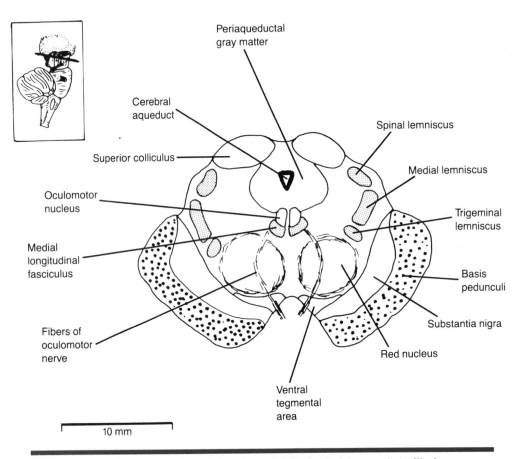

Periaqueductal
gray matter

Cerebral
aqueduct

Spinal lemniscus

Superior colliculus

Medial lemniscus

Oculomotor
nucleus

Trigeminal
lemniscus

Medial
longitudinal
fasciculus

Basis
pedunculi

Substantia nigra

Fibers of
oculomotor
nerve

Red nucleus

Ventral
tegmental
area

10 mm

Figure 8-8   Transverse section through the midbrain at the level of the superior colliculus.

Chapter 9

The Cerebellum

The cerebellum is a large part of the brain, essential for the production of coordinated movements. It consists of two **hemispheres** and a midline portion, the **vermis,** which joins the hemispheres dorsally.

General Organization

Most of the neurons of the cerebellum are in the **cortex** of the external surface, which has a large area because it is greatly folded and fissured. The convexities are known in the cerebellum as **folia** (singular, *folium*). The folia and intervening grooves are mostly horizontally aligned. There is a large core of white matter, consisting of axons going to and from the cortex. Embedded in the white matter are three pairs of **cerebellar nuclei.**

The cerebellum is connected with the brain stem by three large bundles of myelinated axons, the **cerebellar peduncles,** on each side. The inferior cerebellar peduncle is joined to the medulla, the middle peduncle (the largest) is joined to the pons, and the superior peduncle is joined to the midbrain.

Every afferent axon coming into the cerebellum gives off a branch to one of the nuclei and then goes on to terminate in the cortex. The afferent fibers are *excitatory* at their synapses. The output of the cerebellar cortex consists of axons that end in the nuclei, at *inhibitory* synapses. Neurons in the cerebellar nuclei give rise to all the efferent axons that leave the cerebellum. Thus the afferent connections of the cerebellum "drive" its nuclei, but the output of the nuclei is subject to inhibitory control by the cortex (Fig. 9-1).

The cytoarchitecture and internal neuronal circuitry of the cerebellar cortex are uniform throughout the cerebellum. There are three layers: The **molecular layer** consists largely of neurites and snyapses; it lies immediately beneath the pia mater covering the surface of the cortex. The **Purkinje cell layer** is only one cell thick; it consists of the large, evenly spaced Purkinje* cells. These neurons have their richly branched dendritic trees in the molecular layer. Their axons pass through the granular layer and the white matter, to end in the cerebellar nuclei. The **granular layer** consists of interneurons, the granule cells, and their afferent synapses. The intracortical circuitry is shown in simplified form in Figure 9-2.

The major features of cerebellar cortical circuitry are as follows:

1. There are 3 types of afferent fibers. **Climbing fibers** all come from the inferior olivary complex of nuclei of the medulla. These nuclei are influenced by afferents from the cerebral cortex, the spinal cord, and the red nucleus of the midbrain. Climbing fibers are thought to be the source of programs of instructions that are remem-

---

* JE Purkinje (1787–1869) was a Czechoslovakian histologist. He also described the specialized cardiac muscle fibers that are named after him.

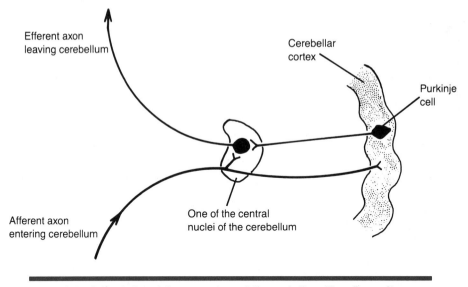

Figure 9-1   General plan of the connections of the cerebellum. The afferent fibers are excitatory; the Purkinje cells, which provide the sole output of the cortex, are inhibitory to the neurons of the cerebellar nuclei.

bered in the cerebellum. The "instructions" are eventually delivered to the parts of the brain that direct the activities of motor neurons. **Noradrenaline-containing fibers** come from the locus ceruleus. These neurons have axons that go to most parts of the central nervous system (see Chap. 21). The fibers that end in the cerebellum may modulate synaptic activity in the molecular layer of the cortex. **Mossy fibers** are the endings of all the cerebellar afferent fibers other than those from the inferior olive or the locus ceruleus. Mossy fibers are thought to be involved in the execution of programms of instructions and in their modification while movements are being carried out.

2.   The number of cortical neurons is much greater than the numbers of afferent fibers and of neurons in the cerebellar nuclei. This large amount of cortex is consistent with its role as a storehouse of information with the associated connec-

tions needed for depositing, recalling, and changing programs.

3.   The sole output of the cerebellar cortex is the axons of the GABAergic Purkinje cells, which inhibit the neurons of the cerebellar nuclei.

Parts of the Cerebellum

Many names have been given to the fissures and groups of folia of the vermis and hemispheres. The few that have significance as anatomical landmarks are indicated in Figure 9-3. This figure also shows the functional divisions of the cerebellum, which are based on the afferent and efferent connections. There are three functional divisions:

1.   **The vestibulocerebellum** consists of the flocculus, the nodule, and parts of the vermis near the nodule. Afferent fibers come from the *ipsilateral* vestibular nu-

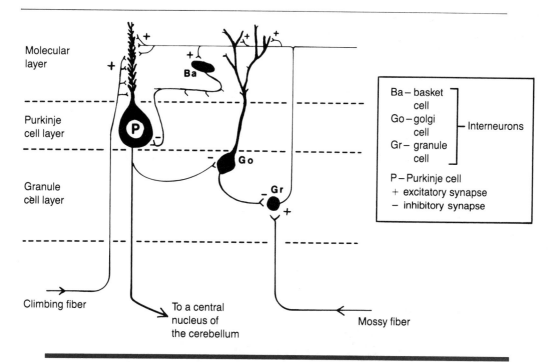

Figure 9-2 The circuitry of the cerebellar cortex arrayed along the long axis of a folium. The large, flattened dendritic trees of the Purkinje cells are spread out across the folium so that each granule cell axon contacts many Purkinje cells. The basket cell axons are directed across the folium, each contacting the axonal hillocks of several Purkinje cells. The dendritic trees of the Golgi cells are spread out in three dimensions. The synaptic complexes in the granule cell layer are known as glomeruli. The pattern of cellular organization is the same throughout the cerebellar cortex. (In contrast, there is great regional variation in the cellular architecture of the cerebral cortex.)

clei in the medulla, and some come directly from the vestibular ganglion. These axons enter the cerebellum through its inferior peduncle. The Purkinje cells in the cortex of the vestibulocerebellum project to the **fastigial nuclei,** which lie close to the midline in the roof of the fourth ventricle (Latin, *fastigium,* meaning roof). The axons of cells in the fastigial nucleus go through the inferior cerebellar peduncle to the vestibular nuclei of *both* sides. (They are accompanied by some axons of Purkinje cells of the vestibulocerebellar cortex, the only exception to the general rule that the cerebellar cortex projects to the cerebellar nuclei.)

2. **The spinocerebellum** consists of the vermis and adjoining cortex of the anterior lobe and of the caudal part of the posterior lobe. These areas are the sites of termination of most of the axons of the spinocerebellar tracts that originate from cell-bodies on the *same side* of the spinal gray matter. Smaller numbers of spinocerebellar fibers are distributed to the lateral parts of the hemispheres. The **dorsal spinocerebellar** tract consists of rapidly conducting axons of cells in the thoracic

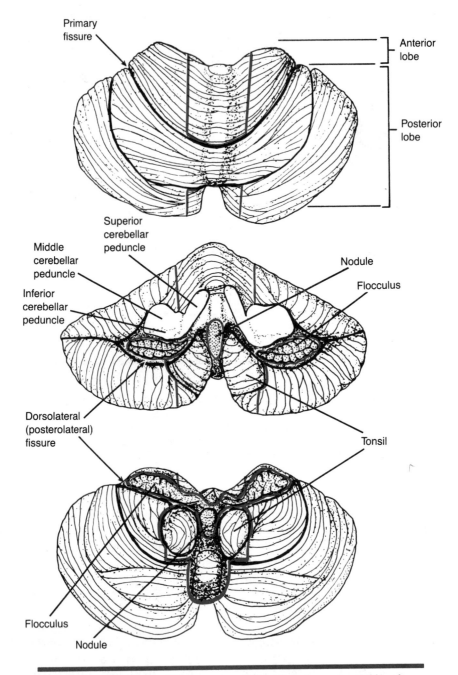

Figure 9-3 The surfaces of the human cerebellum: Superior or dorsal (*Above*); anterior or ventral (*Middle*); inferior or caudal (*Below*). The cerebellum has been removed by cutting its peduncles. Colored lines delineate the functional divisions: **Vestibulocerebellum** (spotted); **spinocerebellum** (unspotted median and medial areas); **pontocerebellum** (lateral to colored lines, and also the vermis of much of the posterior lobe).

nucleus (see Chap. 7), relaying proprioceptive signals from the lower limb. Equivalent fibers for the upper limb arise from the accessory cuneate nucleus of the medulla and constitute the **cuneocerebellar tract.**

The cortex of each paravermal zone projects to the **interposed nucleus** (composed, in man, of the globose and emboliform nuclei), which is lateral to the fastigial nucleus and medial to the dentate nucleus (see below). The neurons in the interposed nucleus send their axons into the superior cerebellar peduncle. The fibers cross the midline in the midbrain and go to the ventral lateral nucleus of the *contralateral* thalamus. This thalamic nucleus projects to the primary motor area of the cerebral cortex. In animals, large numbers of axons from the interposed nucleus synapse with neurons in the red nucleus; it is not known if this connection exists in the human brain.

3. **The pontocerebellum** is the largest functional division. It consists of the lateral parts of the hemispheres and the vermis of much of the posterior lobe. The afferent fibers are the axons of the neurons of the *contralateral* pontine nuclei. They decussate in the basilar (ventral) part of the

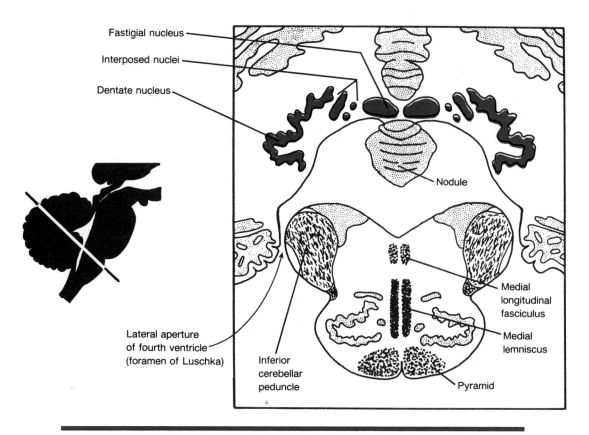

Figure 9-4 A transverse section through the brain stem and cerebellum showing the positions of the cerebellar nuclei.

pons and then form the middle cerebellar peduncle. Purkinje cell axons from the pontocerebellar cortex terminate in the **dentate nucleus** (Fig. 9-4), the largest and most lateral of the cerebellar nuclei. The axons of the dentate neurons accompany those of the cells of the interposed nucleus through the superior cerebellar peduncle, across the midline in the midbrain, to the *contralateral* ventral lateral nucleus of the thalamus.

The afferent cerebellar connections that specify the three functional divisions all end as mossy fibers in the cortex. In addition, there are climbing fibers from the contralateral inferior olivary complex of nuclei that enter the cerebellum through its inferior peduncle and go to all parts of the cortex. The olivary complex is influenced by the cerebral cortex, the red nucleus, and the spinal cord.

Connections and Functions

The connections of the cerebellum with the rest of the central nervous system are de-scribed in Chapter 24. The following points are noteworthy:

1. Each hemicerebellum is connected, directly or indirectly, with the parts of the central nervous system that serve the *same side of the body,* that is, with the contralateral cerebral hemisphere, and with the ipsilateral spinal gray matter.

2. The parts of the cerebellum in and near the midline are concerned principally with the axial muscles and with the maintenance of an upright posture. The lateral parts of the hemispheres are concerned with movements involving the ends of the limbs.

3. The cerebellum ensures that muscles contract at the right times and with the right amount of force to produce the right amount of movement. Disorders of cerebellar function are therefore attributable to lack of coordination of time, force, and duration of muscular contractions. These disorders are discussed in Chapter 24, along with other non-paralyzing disorders of movement.

Chapter 10

The Diencephalon

Parts and Their Locations

The diencephalon has four parts. The largest is the **thalamus.*** There is a thalamus on each side of the slit-like third ventricle. Each is shaped like an egg, with the small end pointing forwards and somewhat medially. In naming the parts of the thalamus, the adjectives "anterior" and "posterior" are used, rather than "rostral" and "caudal." The **hypothalamus** is ventral to the thalamus, forming the floor and lower parts of the walls of the third ventricle. The **subthalamus** is lateral and dorsal to the hypothalamus, so it is not in contact with the ventricular system. **The epithalamus** is dorsal to the thalamus, where the third ventricle becomes the cerebral aqueduct. Although the third ventricle is the cavity of the diencephalon, the thalamus also forms the floor of the lateral ventricle.

The parts of the diencephalon are best appreciated by dissecting the brain and examining sections cut in the coronal (transverse) and horizontal planes. Figure 10-1 shows simplified drawings of representative sections. The *internal capsule,* which bounds the diencephalon laterally, is an important body of nerve fibers going to and from the cerebral cortex. The *fornix,* which forms the roof of the third ventricle, is part of the limbic system. Figure 10-1 also shows the *choroid plexus,* which secretes the cerebrospinal fluid into the lateral and third ventricles. The optic nerves and retinas develop as outgrowths from the diencephalon. Most of the axons of the human optic nerves end in the lateral geniculate bodies of the thalami.

Thalamus

The thalamus exhibits the following gross anatomical features. The **anterior tubercle** (at the pointed end of the "egg") contains the anterior group of nuclei. The expanded posterior end of the thalamus is the **pulvinar** (from the Latin for "cushion"). Ventral to the pulvinar are the **lateral** and **medial geniculate bodies,** containing important nuclei of the auditory and visual systems, respectively. On the medial surface, which is also the wall of the third ventricle, there is usually a body of gray matter that forms a bridge across the third ventricle, connecting the two thalami. Dorsal to this is a longitudinal ridge, the **stria medullaris thalami,** which is a tract connected with the epithalamus.

Internally, the thalamus is divided by the **internal medullary lamina,** a vertical partition

---

* From Greek and Latin words meaning an inner room of a house. The name was first used by the Roman physician Claudius Galen (131–201), who said the optic nerves and tracts were hollow and that each originated from a cavity within the cerebral hemisphere. Although Galen probably had the lateral ventricle in mind, later scholars, notably Thomas Willis (see also Chap. 29), used "thalamus" for the solid region that includes the destination of most of the fibers of the optic tract.

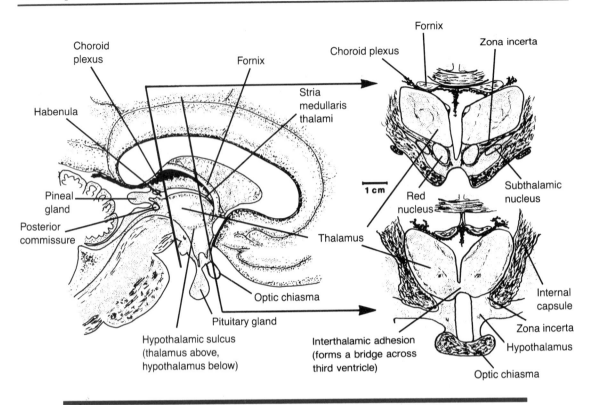

Figure 10-1   Two sections (on right) through the human diencephalon. The picture on the left shows the medial surface of a brain that has been cut in half in the midline to reveal the parts of the diencephalon that form the wall of the third ventricle. Ruled lines indicate the planes of the two transverse (coronal) sections.

of white matter that splits anteriorly to enclose the anterior nuclear group. The internal medullary lamina also splits to enclose the intralaminar nuclei, in the middle of the thalamus. Lateral to the bulk of the thalamus is the **external medullary lamina,** and lateral (to this is the sheet-like reticular nucleus of the thalamus.

The nuclei of the thalamus are named according to their positions. The most important ones are shown in Figure 10-2. Thalamic nuclei are central to many systems of functional connections in the brain. Table 10-1, which summarizes the major connections of the thalamus, is provided for reference. Thalamic

connections provide a useful focus for revising one's knowledge of neural circuitry.

The ventral limit of the thalamus is marked by a groove, the **hypothalamic sulcus,** in the wall of the third ventricle. Anteriorly, the hypothalamus is continuous with the **preoptic area,** which includes the lamina terminalis joining the optic chiasma to the anterior commissure. The preoptic area is, strictly speaking, part of the telencephalon. Laterally, the hypothalamus is bounded by the internal capsule, and posteriorly it becomes continuous with the tegmentum of the midbrain.

The hypothalamus contains many named nuclei. The functions of most of the individual

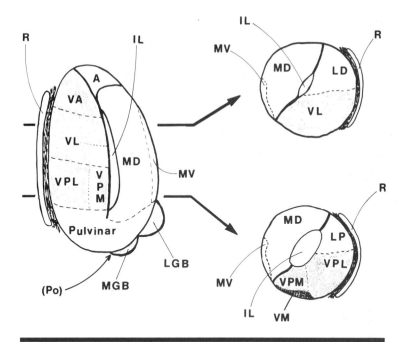

Figure 10-2 Diagram to show the nuclear groups of the thalamus. On the left, the left thalamus is sectioned horizontally and viewed from above. Arrows indicate the levels of the two transverse (coronal) sections, which are of the right thalamus viewed from behind. *Abbreviations are explained in Table 10-1.* The **VL** has anterior and posterior divisions. The **VPL** and **VPM** are divisions of the same (**VP**) nucleus. The black line of white matter that splits to enclose the **IL** nuclei is the **internal medullary lamina.** The **external medullary lamina** intervenes between the reticular nucleus (**R**) and the main mass of the thalamus. The **Po** nuclei and the **geniculate bodies** are beneath (ventral, or inferior to) the **pulvinar.**

nuclei are but poorly understood, however, so it is easier to divide the hypothalamus into larger regions (Fig. 10-3). The **anterior hypothalamus** is dorsal to the optic chiasma. The **tuberal region** comprises the tuber cinereum, the median lump from which the stalk of the pituitary gland arises. The **median eminence** is the site at which the stalk attaches to the tuber cinereum. The **posterior hypothalamus** consists of the **mammillary bodies,** together with more dorsally placed groups of neurons.

The lateral part of the hypothalamus contains great numbers of rostrocaudally aligned nerve fibers, which constitute the **medial forebrain bundle.** This bundle contains axons connecting the hypothalamus with the septal area of the forebrain and with the tegmentum of the midbrain. The other tracts connected with the hypothalamus are the **fornix** (from the hippocampal formation), the **stria terminalis** (from the amygdala), the **dorsal longitudinal fasciculus** (connecting hypothalamus with brain stem and spinal cord), the **mammillothalamic tract** (going to the anterior thalamic nuclei), the **mammillotegmental tract** (going to the midbrain), and the efferents to the pituitary

Table 10-1. Thalamic Nuclei and Their Connections

(Positions of the nuclei are shown in Fig. 10-2. The names of the best understood nuclei are in **bold type.**)

Thalamic Nucleus (or group of nuclei)	Sources of Afferent Fibers	Reciprocal Cortical Connections
	Ventral Group of Nuclei	
Medial geniculate body (MGB)	Inferior colliculus	Auditory cortex of temporal lobe
Lateral geniculate body (LGB)	Retina (through optic tract)	Visual cortex of occipital lobe
Ventral posterior nucleus (VP) **Lateral part (VPL)**	Spinal cord (via spinothalamic tract); gracile & cuneate nuclei (via medial lemniscus)	Primary somatosensory area (postcentral gyrus of parietal lobe)
Medial part (VPM)	Trigeminal sensory nuclei (through trigeminal lemniscus)	
Ventral lateral nucleus (VL)	Cerebellar nuclei Globus pallidus	Primary motor area Premotor area
Ventral anterior nucleus (VA)	(Not known)	Probably to many cortical areas
Principal ventral medial (VMp) nucleus	Spinal cord and substantia nigra	Frontal lobe and cingulate gyrus
Ventral medial basal nucleus (VM$_b$)	Parabrachial nucleus	Gustatory area
	Posterior Group of Nuclei	
Posterior (Po) group	Spinal cord; tectum	Cortex of and around insula
	Medial Group of Nuclei	
Mediodorsal (MD) (dorsomedial) **nucleus**	Amygdala, hypothalamus, and olfactory cortex	Frontal lobe (including orbitofrontal cortex)
Medioventral nucleus (MV) (nucleus reuniens)	Parts of parahippocampal and cingulate gyri	Entohinal area and hippocampus
	Anterior Group of Nuclei	
Anterior nuclei (Ant)	Mammillary body	Cingulate gyrus
	Lateral Group of Nuclei	
Lateral dorsal nucleus (LD)	Hippocampus	Cingulate gyrus
Lateral posterior nucleus (LP)	(Not known)	Association areas of parietal lobe
Nuclei of the pulvinar (Plv)	Superior colliculus; pretectal area; retina	Parietal, temporal, and occipital lobes
	Intralaminar Group of Nuclei	
Intralaminar nuclei (IL)	Spinal cord; reticular formation; also other regions	Parietal and frontal lobes; caudate nucleus and putamen
	Reticular Nucleus of Thalamus	
Reticular nucleus (R)	Receives branches of all thalamocortical and corticothalamic axons. Axons of cells in R end within all other thalamic nuclei	

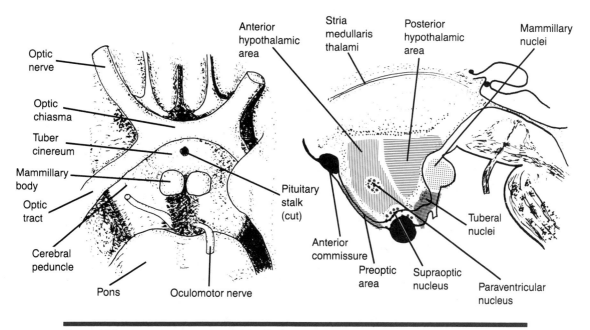

Figure 10-3 Ventral surface of the brain (*Left*) showing parts of the hypothalamus. The section (*Right*) is a little to the right of the midline to show the groups of hypothalamic nuclei.

gland, described in the next section of this chapter.

The Hypophysis or Pituitary Gland

The hypophysis develops from both the neural tube and the endoderm of the pharynx. A ventral growth from the diencephalon meets Rathke's pouch, a dorsal outgrowth of the pharynx.* The adult gland consequently contains central nervous tissue (the **neurohypophysis**) and ordinary endocrine glandular tissue (the **adenohypophysis**).

The neurohypophysis has two parts, the **median eminence** (which can also be considered as part of the tuber cinereum of the hypo-

*Martin Heinrich Rathke (1793–1860) was a German scientist who made important contributions to anatomy, physiology, zoology, and pathology.

thalamus), and the **posterior lobe.** These are connected by the **pituitary stalk,** which consists largely of the unmyelinated axons of neurosecretory cells in the supraoptic and paraventricular nuclei. The median eminence and posterior lobe are neurohemal organs, where the products of neurosecretory cells are stored in axonal terminals, and released into the blood. The largest part of the adenohypophysis is the **anterior lobe.**

The nomenclature of the hypophysis is quite complicated, and many names are used to specify the different parts accurately. These are summarized in Figure 10-4.

The Epithalamus

This part of the diencephalon consists of three structures.

1. The **pineal gland** (so named because it is shaped like a pine cone), or **epiphysis cer-**

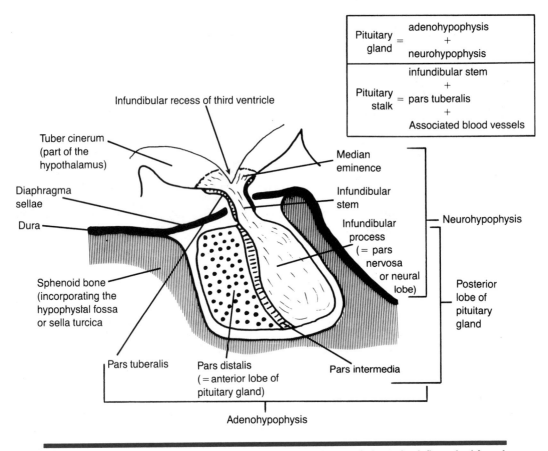

Pituitary gland	=	adenohypophysis + neurohypophysis
Pituitary stalk	=	infundibular stem + pars tuberalis + Associated blood vessels

Infundibular recess of third ventricle

Tuber cinerum (part of the hypothalamus)

Diaphragma sellae

Dura

Sphenoid bone (incorporating the hypophystal fossa or sella turcica

Median eminence

Infundibular stem

Infundibular process (= pars nervosa or neural lobe)

Neurohypophysis

Posterior lobe of pituitary gland

Pars tuberalis

Pars distalis (= anterior lobe of pituitary gland)

Pars intermedia

Adenohypophysis

Figure 10-4   Sagittal (midline) section through the hypothalamus, pituitary gland (hypophysis), and base of skull. The labeling explains the nomenclature of the parts of the hypophysis. (*Sella turcica* is Latin for "Turkish saddle.")

ebri, develops around an outgrowth of the third ventricle, dorsal to the point at which the cerebral aqueduct leaves the ventricle. The short, hollow stalk of the gland is attached to the left and right habenulae.

2. The **habenula** of each side consists of medial and lateral habenular nuclei. Afferent fibers come to the habenula in the stria medullaris thalami. The habenulae are connected by a small habenular commissure, in the dorsal part of the pineal stalk. The connections of the habenular nuclei

form part of the limbic system. In Latin, *habenula* means a little strap.

3. The **posterior commissure,** in the ventral part of the pineal stalk, is also included in the epithalamus, though it consists of axons of mesencephalic neurons involved in movements of the eyes and pupils.

The Pineal Gland

The characteristic cells of the gland are **pinealocytes,** which are derived from the neural tube and might be classified as specialized neurons or glial cells. The gland also contains astrocytes and blood vessels. The pinealocytes secrete **melatonin,** an indole amine formed by enzymatic transformation of serotonin. The pinealocytes are innervated by noradrenergic postganglionic sympathetic fibers from the superior cervical ganglion. Although the pineal gland is attached to the habenulae, it probably does not receive axons from the central nervous system in mammals.

The best known pharmacological action of melatonin is its granule-aggregating action on the melanophores of amphibian skin, which becomes pale in response to the hormone. This action opposes the melanotrophic hormone of the pars intermedia of the adenohypophysis, which disperses the melanin granules and thereby darkens the skin. No comparable control of color exists in mammals, which do not have cells equivalent to the melanophores of lower vertebrates.

In some mammals the secretion of melatonin fluctuates with ambient illumination, both in the day/night cycle and with the seasons of the year. The control mechanism involves retinal neurons whose axons end in the hypothalamus, and hypothalamic neurons that project to preganglionic sympathetic neurons. The pineal gland forms a necessary link between the eyes and the hypothalamo–hypophysial system in the timing of the reproductive cycles of seasonally breeding animals. There is also evidence for an "antigonadotrophic" influence of the pineal gland in prepubertal animals.

In fishes and amphibians, the epiphysis contains photoreceptor cells that respond to light perceived through the overlying skin and bone. These receptors are connected with the optic tectum (see Chap. 12) and may be involved in the endocrine mechanisms controlling skin color and reproductive cycles. In some lizards, there is a well-developed dorsal median photoreceptor organ, the parietal eye. This is an outgrowth from the telencephalon,

however, and is not homologous with the epiphysis.

The functions of the human pineal gland are unknown. From about the 30th year, increasing quantities of calcareous material ("pineal sand") accumulate within the astrocytes, so the gland becomes a useful radiographic marker of the midline.

The pineal gland rests on the dorsum of the midbrain, above and between the superior colliculi. Pressure from a tumor of the gland causes paralysis of upward gaze and may obstruct the flow of cerebrospinal fluid through the cerebral aqueduct.

The Subthalamus

The **subthalamic nucleus** (see Fig. 10-1) is involved, together with the corpus striatum, in the control of movement.

The other regions of gray matter in the subthalamus are the rostral poles of the substantia nigra and red nucleus (nuclei of the midbrain), and the **zona incerta,** a group of neurons placed between the lateral hypothalamus and the ventral edge of the thalamic reticular nucleus. Functionally, the zona incerta is associated with the hypothalamus in the control of drinking behavior.

The remaining components of the subthalamus are bundles of myelinated axons about to enter the ventral nuclei of the thalamus. The **prerubral field** consists of the preterminal parts of three ascending sensory tracts, the medial, spinal, and trigeminal lemnisci, and the dentatothalamic fibers from the cerebellum. The prerubral field is also known as "field H of Forel."* The "H" is from the German *Haube,* a cap. Fields H_1 and H_2 of Forel are bundles of **pallidothalamic fibers** passing through the subthalamus as they go from the medial part of the corpus striatum to the thalamus.

* AH Forel: See footnote in Chapter 13.

Chapter 11

The Telencephalon

The two cerebral hemispheres rostral to the thalami constitute the telencephalon. The cavity of each hemisphere is the lateral ventricle. The large masses of telencephalic gray matter in and close to the lateral wall of the lateral ventricle constitute the **corpus striatum.** External to the corpus striatum is the medullary center of the hemisphere, the **cerebral white matter.** On the outside surface is another layer of gray matter, the **cerebral cortex.** The olfactory tract and olfactory bulb, attached to the ventral surface, arise as an outgrowth of the embryonic telencephalon, but in the adult state the cavity has been obliterated. The **septal area** is a small region on the medial surface of the hemisphere, rostral to the hypothalamus.

Chapter 12 contains a brief account of the comparative anatomy of the telencephalon. There the reader will see that the gray masses constituting the septum, the corpus striatum, and the pallium (cerebral cortex and related structures) are evolved from different parts of the walls of a simple tubular hemisphere. In the human brain, however, the lateral ventricle is not tubular, but C-shaped, usually with a small posterior appendage to the middle part of the "C." The gray and white matter are arrayed around this ventricle, whose shape provides the cerebral hemisphere with five **lobes**—the frontal, parietal, occipital, temporal, and insular lobes. The first four lobes are named after the overlying bones of the skull. The insular lobe (or simply "insula") is in the floor of the deep lateral sulcus that separates the temporal from the parietal and frontal lobes.

Cerebral Cortex

The cortex has many named grooves (**sulci,** singular *sulcus*) and convexities (**gyri,** singular *gyrus*). Only a few are important as anatomical landmarks or because of known functions. They are illustrated in Figure 11-1.

Several *functional areas* are also recognized within the cerebral cortex. These are discussed, together with the cellular architecture and common disorders of the cortex, in Chapter 22.

Cerebral White Matter

The medullary center of the cerebral hemisphere consists of interlacing bundles of nerve fibers of three types—association, commissural, and projection fibers.

Association fibers may be short, connecting areas of cortex in the same or adjacent gyri or sulci, or long, connecting more distant areas. Many of the long association fibers are in named bundles that can be revealed by blunt dissection. Association bundles connect the cortex of every lobe of the hemisphere with that of every other lobe. The list in Table 11-1 is provided for reference.

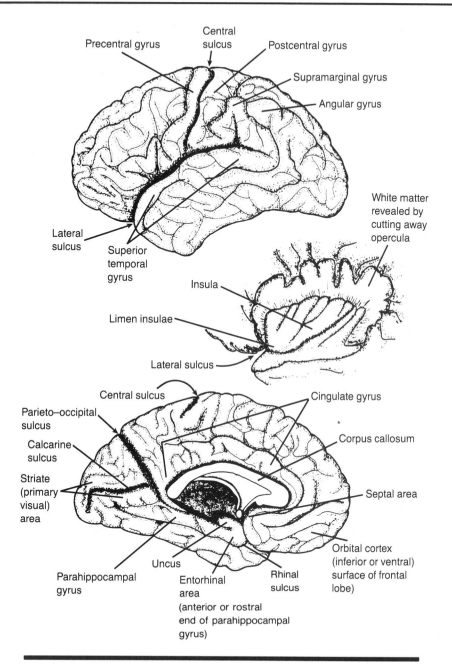

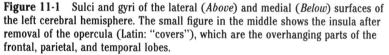

Figure 11-1 Sulci and gyri of the lateral (*Above*) and medial (*Below*) surfaces of the left cerebral hemisphere. The small figure in the middle shows the insula after removal of the opercula (Latin: "covers"), which are the overhanging parts of the frontal, parietal, and temporal lobes.

Table 11-1.   Association Bundles

Name	Areas Connected
Superior longitudinal (arcuate) fasciculus	Frontal lobe to occipital and temporal lobes
Superior occipitofrontal fasciculus (or subcallosal bundle)	Frontal lobe to occipital lobe
Inferior occipitofrontal fasciculus	Frontal lobe to occipital lobe
Uncinate fasciculus	Frontal lobe to temporal lobe
Inferior longitudinal fasciculus	Occipital lobe to temporal lobe
Cingulum	Cingulate gyrus to parahippocampal gyrus
Fornix (not in the medullary center)	Hippocampal formation to septal area, thalamus and hypothalamus

Commissural fibers connect symmetrical areas of the cortices of the two hemispheres. These fibers form two bundles, both compact and conspicuous in the midline, but more diffuse laterally. The **corpus callosum** is the larger commissure. In the midline it consists of a **rostrum** (Latin for "beak") rostrally, a **splenium** (from the Greek for "bandage," though it does not look like one) caudally, and a **trunk** in between. The name *corpus callosum* means "hard body" in Latin, making reference to the tough consistency of this large sheet of white matter. On each side of the midline, the corpus callosum forms most of the roof of the lateral ventricle. In the midline, the **septum pellucidum** is attached to the ventral surface of the corpus callosum. The septum pellucidum is a double membrane, made largely of neuroglia, which separates the left lateral ventricle from the right. The ventral edge of the septum pellucidum is attached to the body of the fornix, which is the roof of the third ventricle. The **anterior commissure** is much smaller than the corpus callosum. It connects the cortices of the temporal lobes and also contains some decussating fibers of the olfactory system.

Holes in the septum pellucidum occur regularly in professional boxers, but are not believed to give rise to symptoms. The septum is a useful radiological marker of the midline. Occasionally cysts develop within the septum and press on nearby structures.

The splenium of the corpus callosum is larger in women than in men, but it is not known how this difference relates to the functions of the cerebral commissures, which are discussed in Chapter 22.

Projection fibers go to and from the cerebral cortex. They form distinct bundles only around the thalamus and corpus striatum. The most important aggregation of projection fibers is the **internal capsule,** at the base of the cerebral hemisphere. Lesions in the internal capsule cause serious disability because many important connections are concentrated in a small area.

The internal capsule is bounded medially by the thalamus and by part of the corpus striatum, the head of the caudate nucleus. Another component of the corpus striatum, the lentiform nucleus, is lateral to the internal capsule. The fibers communicating with the cortex of the temporal lobe pass beneath the lentiform nucleus. Figure 11-2 shows the an-

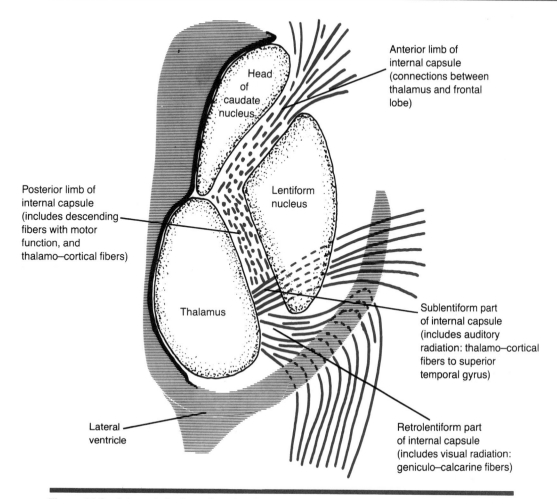

Anterior limb of
internal capsule
(connections between
thalamus and frontal
lobe)

Head
of
caudate
nucleus

Lentiform
nucleus

Posterior limb of
internal capsule
(includes descending
fibers with motor
function, and
thalamo–cortical fibers)

Thalamus

Sublentiform part
of internal capsule
(includes auditory
radiation: thalamo–cortical
fibers to superior
temporal gyrus)

Lateral
ventricle

Retrolentiform part
of internal capsule
(includes visual radiation:
geniculo–calcarine fibers)

Figure 11-2   Schematic horizontal section through the right lateral ventricle, thalamus, and corpus striatum, showing the parts of the internal capsule.

atomical relations and the parts of the internal capsule.

Corpus Striatum and Basal Ganglia

The corpus striatum consists of the **caudate** and **lentiform nuclei,** in the cerebral hemisphere. The name "striped body" refers to the visible fasciculi of myelinated axons in these large masses of gray matter. The term "basal ganglia" includes the corpus striatum, the subthalamic nucleus of the diencephalon, and the substantia nigra of the midbrain. All these nuclei are involved in the control of movement.

The anatomical terminology of the corpus striatum is rather complicated; it is explained in the following summary.

Lentiform { Globus pallidus   = Pallidum = Paleostriatum
nucleus   { Putamen
            Caudate nucleus } = Striatum = Neostriatum

It can be seen that there are two functional components of the corpus striatum: the pallidum or paleostriatum, and the striatum or neostriatum. Although the caudate and lentiform nuclei have different names, they are fused anteriorly, where the head of the caudate nucleus becomes continuous with the putamen.

The anatomy of the corpus striatum and of the internal capsule are best learned by dissecting the brain or examining models. It is also necessary to be familiar with the structures present in a horizontal section of the cerebral hemisphere passing through the insula (Fig. 11-3).

Other structures inside the cerebral hemisphere are the **claustrum** (about which very little is known), the **external capsule** (consisting of corticostriatal and probably other projection fibers), and the **extreme capsule,** which probably consists largely of fibers going to and from the cortex of the insula. The **substantia innominata** is between the hypothalamus and the ventral surface of the temporal lobe. The **anterior perforated substance** is at the caudal end of the olfactory tract, and the **septal area,** below the rostrum of the corpus callosum, is part of the limbic system.

Temporal Lobe

The temporal lobe contains the lower limb of the C-shaped lateral ventricle. Most of the

Frontal pole of hemisphere

Corpus callosum
(anterior or rostral end)

Head of caudate nucleus

Putamen ⎫
            ⎬ Lentiform
Globus   ⎪ nucleus
pallidus   ⎭

External capsule

Internal capsule

Claustrum

Cortex of insula

Thalamus

Lateral ventricle

Fornix

Corpus callosum
(posterior or caudal end)

Occipital pole of hemisphere

5 cm

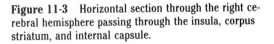

Figure 11-3 Horizontal section through the right cerebral hemisphere passing through the insula, corpus striatum, and internal capsule.

surface of the temporal lobe is covered by cortex similar to that of the other lobes of the cerebrum, but the medial side of the ventral (inferior) surface of the temporal cortex, the parahippocampal gyrus, is composed of a different type of cortex and is part of the limbic system. The cortex medial to the parahippocampal gyrus is rolled inwards so that it comes to lie inside the temporal lobe, there to form the floor of the lateral ventricle. This internal cortical mass, which is also part of the limbic system, is the **hippocampus.** This name is from the Greek for "sea-horse," but the resemblance of the cerebral structure to the fish is not at all obvious. The **fornix** is a large tract leading dorsally and medially out of the caudal (posterior) end of the hippocampus and forming part of the medial wall of the lateral ventricle.

The caudate nucleus is shaped like a tadpole, with its large head in the frontal lobe and its tail following the curve of the lateral ventricle into the temporal lobe. The end of the tail of the caudate nucleus is in contact with the **amygdala** (or amygdaloid body), a group of nuclei immediately beneath the cortex of the **uncus,** which is the most medial part of the parahippocampal gyrus. The name *amygdala* is Latin for "almond" and reasonably approximates its size and shape. The connections of the amygdaloid nuclei are with the olfactory and limbic systems.

Some of the anatomical features of the temporal lobe are best appreciated in a transverse (coronal) section through the cerebral hemisphere (Fig. 11-4), which also shows the corpus striatum, the internal capsule, and parts of the lateral ventricle.

Lateral Ventricle

Knowledge of the anatomy of the lateral ventricle helps in understanding the topography of the neural components of the telencephalon and diencephalon. Furthermore, the ventricular system is displayed in special diagnostic x-ray pictures of the brain, so that the clinician may detect abnormalities of size or shape due to disease.

As stated earlier, each lateral ventricle is roughly C-shaped. The **central part** of the ventricle is in the upper part of the curve, and it extends into the frontal lobe as the **frontal horn** (also called "anterior horn"). The long lower part of the ventricle is the **temporal horn** (also called "inferior horn"), which extends into the temporal lobe. The **occipital horn** (or "posterior horn") varies greatly in size and is occasionally absent. It extends from the central part of the ventricle into the occipital lobe.

The roof of the lateral ventricle is formed largely by the **corpus callosum.** The floor of the central part of the lateral ventricle is the dorsal surface of the **thalamus.** Lateral and anterior to the thalamus is the head of the **caudate nucleus.** The tail of the caudate nucleus follows the curve of the thalamus and of the ventricle and thus comes to lie in the medial part of the roof of the temporal horn. The caudate nucleus and thalamus are separated by a sulcus. A thin bundle of fibers, the **stria terminalis,** is present in the sulcus. The stria terminalis consists of axons originating in the amygdala; they run alongside the tail of the caudate nucleus, then between the head of the caudate nucleus and the thalamus, and finally turn ventrally to end in the septal area and hypothalamus. The **amygdala** indents the tip of the temporal horn.

The medial part of the floor of the temporal horn is formed by the **hippocampus.** The ventricular surface of the hippocampus is made of white matter and is called the **alveus,** a word which, mysteriously, is Latin for "trough." The fibers of the alveus gather together to form a flange, the **fimbria** (Latin for "fringe"), on the medial side of the hippocampus. The fimbria becomes larger posteriorly as it accumulates more fibers, and at the caudal (posterior) end of the hippocampus it becomes the **crus of the fornix.** In Latin, *crus* is

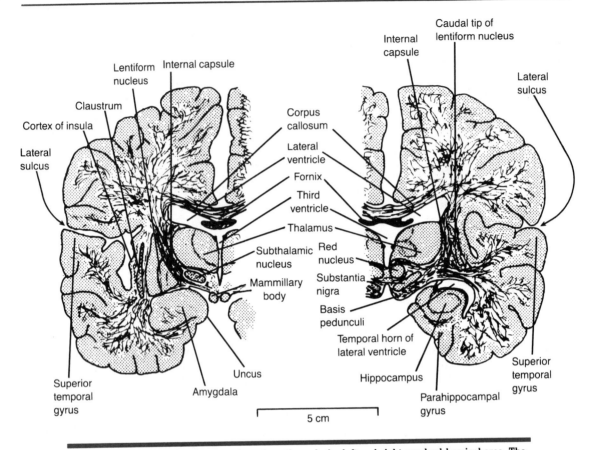

Figure 11-4 Coronal (or transverse) sections through the left and right cerebral hemispheres. The section on the left is about 1.5 cm rostral to the one on the right. (Compare with Figs. 10-1 and 10-3 to locate landmarks on the ventral surface.)

a leg and *fornix* is an arch in a roof; both terms are quite apt. The fornix curves upwards and forwards over the thalamus and then turns ventrally in front of the anterior tubercle of the thalamus. Most of its fibers end in the hypothalamus and septal area. The part of the fornix dorsal to the thalamus is the **body,** and the descending anterior part is the **column.** The bodies of the left and right fornices touch one another, and together form the roof of the third ventricle.

The fornix is separated from the thalamus by the **choroid fissure.** The choroid plexus, which secretes cerebrospinal fluid, protrudes through the choroid fissure into the cavity of the lateral ventricle and also hangs from the roof of the third ventricle. The choroid plexus is supplied by blood vessels that approach the brain from behind by passing under the splenium of the corpus callosum and between the crura of the fornix. Anteriorly, there is an open space between the column of the fornix and the anterior tubercle of the thalamus. This is the **interventricular foramen** of Monro,* through which the cavities of the lateral and third ventricle are in continuity.

* Alexander Monro II (1733–1817) was a professor of anatomy at Edinburgh. He followed his father and was followed by his son. All three incumbents of the chair were called Alexander.

Chapter 12

Comparative Neuroanatomy

It is quite feasible to learn about the human nervous system without knowing anything about the nervous systems of other animals. A comparative approach is helpful, however, in showing the application of some simple principles of structural organization. Thus all nervous systems contain distinct cells, the neurons, that conduct signals and communicate at synapses. Neurons are much the same throughout the animal kingdom. On a larger scale, even the most primitive vertebrate animals have central nervous systems made of parts that are homologous with parts of the human brain and spinal cord.

Invertebrates

The nervous systems of two radially symmetrical animals are shown in Figure 12-1. In the simpler animal, *Hydra,* the neurons have two to five neurites each and are uniformly distributed throughout the body wall. Physical contact at any point causes the cells of the wall to contract and bend toward the stimulus. A food particle in the midst of the tentacles is thus pushed into the mouth, and simple locomotion of the animal is also possible. The contraction of cells remote from the site of stimulation is possible because communication among the neurons of the nerve net is much faster than among ordinary cells. The intensity of the stimulus determines the number of neurons that become active and

thereby dictates the size of the movement. There are no preferred routes of communication within the nervous system of *Hydra.* Coelenterates more advanced than *Hydra,* such as sea anemones and jellyfish, have more complicated nerve nets, with different populations of neurons coordinating different movements, and sometimes with regions that can be designated as ganglia because they are densely populated with neurons. The most advanced radially symmetrical animals are the echinoderms, such as the starfish *Asterias* (Fig. 12-1). In these, as in the coelenterates, there is no tendency toward a single centralized system. The neurons are, however, concentrated into rings and radiating cords.

The simplest animals with bilateral symmetry are the platyhelminths or flatworms, such as the common planarian, *Dugesia* (Fig. 12-2). Flatworms resemble the coelenterates in having a single orifice that serves as mouth and anus. In these animals there is a diffuse nerve net beneath the ectoderm, but neurons are also present in longitudinally running nerve cords. *Dugesia* has two such cords, connected with the superficial nerve net and, through commissures, with one another. At the anterior end of a planarian the nerve cords are enlarged and fused, forming a **cerebral ganglion.** This also receives input from nearby chemosensitive (taste) cells, from the light-sensitive eye-spots, and from a gravity-detecting structure, the statocyst. The cerebral ganglion is the simplest kind of brain. In it,

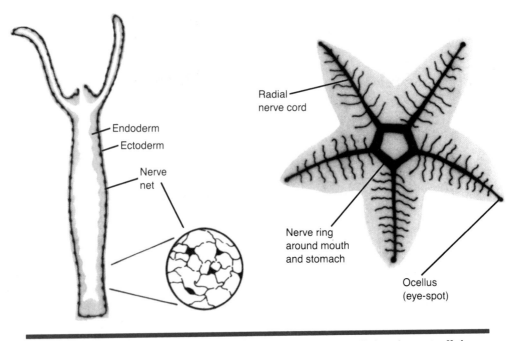

Figure 12-1   Nervous systems of two radially symmetrical animals. (*Left*) A coelenterate, *Hydra*, with a view of part of the nerve-net as seen from the surface. (*Right*) An echinoderm, *Asterias*.

the neuronal cell bodies occupy a peripheral **rind,** and neurites contact one another in the central **core,** in a tissue known as **neuropile.** This rind-and-core structure is seen in the ganglia of all the higher invertebrates too, but not in the nervous systems of vertebrate animals.

The nervous systems of various worms and wormlike animals are shown in Fig. 12-3. These animals all have the mouth and anus widely separated and have well-developed cerebral ganglia around the pharynx and esophagus in what can be unequivocally called a head. Most zoologists think some sort of worm was the ancestor of all vertebrate animals. The currently favorite candidates are the Nemertina or the cephalochordates, or extinct forms resembling these. Less convincing putative ancestors that have been suggested at one time or another include annelids,

scorpionlike arthropods, and even echinoderms.

The invertebrates that exhibit the most elaborate behavior are some of the arthropods and molluscs (see Fig. 12-4). Arthropod nervous systems conform to a general plan, with a brain and one or two ventral nerve cords with segmental ganglia. The nervous systems of molluscs vary greatly in size and complexity, as is to be expected in animals as diverse as clams, snails, and squids. Most behavioral patterns of invertebrates are "hard-wired" into the nervous system. Learning and adaptation are severely restricted by the inadequacy of connections between ganglia in different parts of the body.

The phylum *Chordata* consists of animals in which, at least in some stage of development, there is a tubular cord of nervous tissue dorsal to a skeletal element, the notochord.

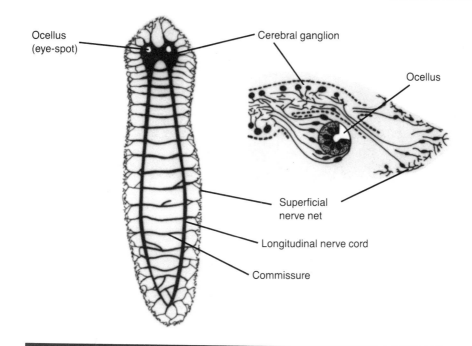

Figure 12-2   Nervous system of *Dugesia*, a planarian flatworm (*Platyhelminthes: Turbellaria*). (*Left*) Dorsal aspect of the whole animal. (The mouth/anus is on the ventral surface.) (*Right*) Section of the anterior end of the animal, in a plane parallel to the midline, showing cerebral ganglion, part of the nerve-net, and an ocellus. The light-sensitive structures are the specialized dendrites of bipolar neurons.

The phylum includes the amphioxus (see Fig. 12-3) and all vertebrate animals.

Vertebrates

All vertebrates have a central nervous system consisting of the brain and spinal cord, protected by the axial skeleton, and a peripheral nervous system consisting of nerves and ganglia (see Fig. 1-1).

Spinal and Cranial Nerves

The **spinal nerves** are segmentally organized. The most primitive vertebrates, the cyclostomes (lampreys and hagfish), have alternating dorsal and ventral spinal nerves. The ventral nerves consist entirely of the axons of neurons in the spinal cord that supply striated skeletal muscle. The dorsal nerves, each with a **spinal ganglion,** contain the axons of neurons in the cord that control viscera together with all sensory axons. A spinal ganglion contains the cell-bodies of sensory neurons, each with a distal neurite distributed in a peripheral nerve and a central neurite that enters the spinal cord.

The dorsal and ventral spinal nerves of cyclostomes correspond in all higher animals to the dorsal and ventral **roots,** which unite to form the mixed spinal nerves. In fishes and amphibians, efferent axons concerned with visceral function leave the spinal cord in the

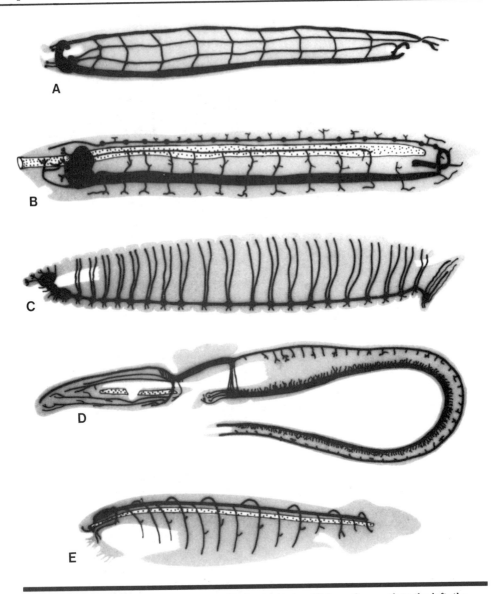

Figure 12-3 Nervous systems of five wormlike invertebrates. All have the mouth to the left, the anus to the right, and the dorsal surface uppermost. Paired nerves are shown only for the left side of each animal. **A.** A nematode or unsegmented roundworm, *Ascaris,* with dorsal and ventral nerve-cords. **B.** A nemertine or ribbonworm (*Neuronemertes*) with a well-developed cerebral ganglion and one dorsal and two ventral nerve-cords. The stippled structure, which is the sheath of the evertible proboscis, is thought by some zoologists to be ancestral to the notochord of vertebrate animals. **C.** An annelid, the leech *Hirudo,* showing well-developed segmentation, with a cerebral ganglion and a ventral ganglionated nerve-cord. **D.** A hemichordate, *Balanoglossus,* with dorsal and ventral nerve-cords and a notochord (stippled) in the proboscis. **E.** A cephalochordate, the amphioxus (*Branchiostoma*), with a notochord (stippled) ventral to the brain and spinal cord, and alternating dorsal and ventral segmental nerves.

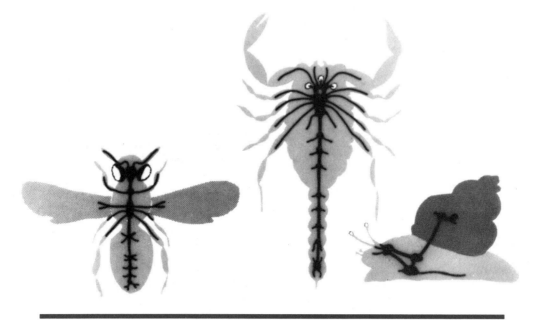

Figure 12-4 Nervous systems of two arthropods, a bee (*Apis*) and a scorpion (*Scorpio*), and of a gastropod mollusc (*Helix*, a snail). Only the ganglia and larger nerves are shown.

ventral and dorsal roots. In reptiles, birds, and mammals, however, there is complete segregation of afferent and efferent nerve fibers.

The **cranial nerves,** which are connected with the brain, have more diverse functions than the spinal nerves. The names, numbers, and functions of the cranial nerves are summarized in Table 12-1. The human cranial nerves are discussed in more detail in other chapters.

Special Sense Organs

Small groups of ectodermally derived sensory cells called **neuromasts** are widespread in the skin of cyclostomes and fishes. In the latter, and also in the aquatic larvae of amphibians, they occupy a system of subcutaneous canals, the **lateral line system.** The canals communicate through pores in the overlying skin with the surrounding water. Lateral line receptors, which are innervated by cranial nerves, detect slow pressure changes (not sounds, which are pressure waves of higher frequency) in the water. In some fishes they also detect electric signals emitted by other fishes. Some of the neuromasts of lampreys are sensitive to light. The sensitivity of neuromasts to radiation and to mechanical stimuli indicates that these sense organs may, in ancestral vertebrates, have evolved into parts of the more advanced special sense organs of higher animals: the inner ear, the taste buds, and the infrared (radiant heat) detecting pits on the heads of some snakes. The olfactory epithelium is thought to have evolved independently of the neuromast system, because it is already well developed in cyclostomes, the most primitive living vertebrates.

Central Nervous System

The **spinal cord** has a hollow core of gray matter surrounded by longitudinally coursing ax-

Table 12-1.   The Cranial Nerves

Number and Name	Principal Functions
I. **Olfactory**	Chemical sensation; gaseous stimuli in land animals (see Chap. 14). The nearby **vomeronasal nerve** (present in most vertebrates, but not in man) detects sniffed or licked liquid chemicals significant in reproduction and territorial marking
II. **Optic**	Vision (see Chap. 18)
III. **Oculomotor**	Supplies the muscles of the eye (except those supplied by IV and VI) and the muscle that elevates the upper eyelid (in animals that have eyelids). Controls visceral functions inside the eye: constriction of pupil and focusing of lens (see Chap. 19)
IV. **Trochlear**	Supplies one eye muscle (the superior oblique, whose tendon passes through the trochlea, a fibrous ring that serves as a pulley [see Chap. 19])
V. **Trigeminal**	Motor to muscles of chewing and a few others near the mouth. Sensory to most of head (Chap. 20) and parts of lateral line system in fishes
VI. **Abducent**	Supplies one eye muscle (the lateral rectus, which abducts the eye [see Chap. 19]). Also supplies muscle of the nictitating membrane ("third eyelid") of reptiles, birds, and some mammals
VII. **Facial**	Motor to muscles of face and a few others. Taste sensation. Controls lacrimal and some salivary glands (see Chap. 20). Serves parts of lateral line system in fishes
VIII. **Vestibulocochlear**	Detection of position and movement. In vertebrates other than fishes, also hearing (see Chaps. 16, 17)
IX. **Glossopharyngeal**	Supplies one muscle of swallowing (the stylopharyngeus). Controls parotid salivary gland. General and taste sensation from pharynx and posterior part of tongue (see Chap. 20). Serves parts of lateral line system in fishes
X. **Vagus**	Motor to muscles of larynx, pharynx, and upper end of esophagus. Controls internal organs, including heart and much of alimentary canal. Several sensory components (see Chap. 20). In fishes, sensory from the lateral line system of the body and tail. The name (Latin for "wandering") indicates the widespread distribution of the nerve's branches. Has also been named the pneumogastric nerve, from branches that go to lungs and stomach.

The last two cranial nerves are absent in all fishes (except the *Crossopterygii,* which are considered by zoologists to be ancestral to limbed vertebrates) and in amphibians. Some fossil amphibians, however, had 12 cranial nerves.

XI. **Accessory**	Motor to some muscles that move the head (see Chap. 20)
XII. **Hypoglossal**	Motor to the muscles of the tongue. (see Chap. 20)

ons. The latter include myelinated fibers in all vertebrates more advanced than cyclostomes. The central canal of the spinal cord expands rostrally into the ventricles of the brain.

The shape of the **brain** (Fig. 12-5) is due partly to the ventricular system and partly to the variable thickness of the nervous tissue forming its walls. As in man, all vertebrates have a hindbrain, midbrain, diencephalon, and telencephalon. In fishes and amphibians, the most conspicuous thickenings are in the left and right sides of the dorsal wall of the midbrain. These constitute the **optic tectum,** which corresponds to the superior colliculus of the human brain. In higher vertebrates, the tectum (Latin for "roof") is relatively smaller. The **cerebellum** is an outgrowth of the dorsal and lateral surfaces of the hindbrain. It is present in all vertebrate groups but is largest in mammals. The optic nerve and the retina of the eye are outgrowths of the **diencephalon.**

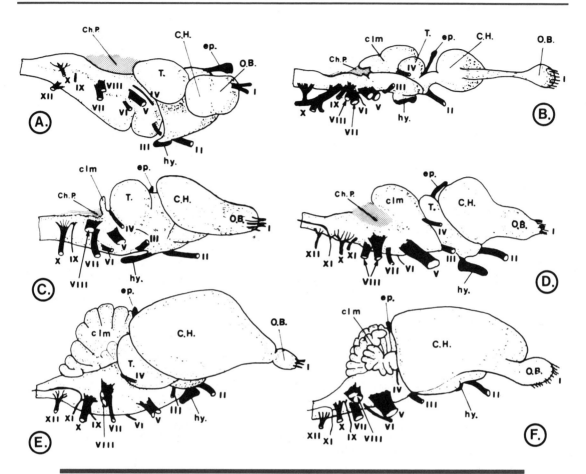

Figure 12-5   Brains of six vertebrate animals: Rostral ends point to the right. (A) A cyclostome (*Lampetra*); (B) A cartilaginous fish (the dogfish, *Squalus*); (C) An amphibian, the frog *Rana;* (D) A reptile, the turtle *Chelone;* (E) A bird, the domestic chicken (*Gallus*); (F) A mammal, the rabbit (*Oryctolagus*). *Abbreviations:* **I–XII** = cranial nerves (see Table 12-1); **C.H.** = cerebral hemisphere; **Ch.P.** = choroid plexus of fourth ventricle; **clm** = cerebellum; **ep.** = epiphysis (= pineal gland); **hy.** = hypophysis (= pituitary gland); **O.B.** = olfactory bulb; **T.** = tectum.

This part of the brain also has two glandular outgrowths: The epiphysis or pineal gland dorsally, and the hypophysis or pituitary gland ventrally.

The size and complexity of the **telencephalon** increase with phylogenetic advancement. The probable homologies of its major parts, the **septum,** the **corpus striatum,** and the **pallium,** are shown in Figure 12-6. The most conspic-

uous part of the human brain is the cerebral cortex: This is the name given to the pallium in mammals.

The variations in structure of the brain among the various mammals are associated with differences in intelligence and in posture. The more intelligent an animal is, the larger is its telencephalon. A quadrupedal animal has its eyes looking along the ground, so its

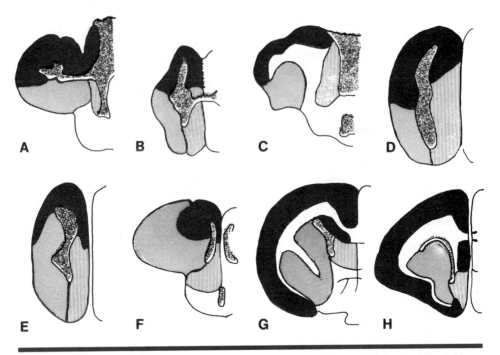

Figure 12-6 Transverse sections through the telencephalon in eight animals, showing the positions and relative sizes of the **septum** (vertical hatching), **corpus striatum** (stippled), and **pallium** (black). The ventricular cavity is colored. (**A**) A cyclostome (*Lampetra*). (**B**) A cartilaginous fish (*Squalus*). (**C**) A bony fish (goldfish, *Carassius*); as in all teleost fishes, the telencephalon is everted, so that a common ventricular cavity with a membranous roof intervenes between left and right sides. (**D**) An amphibian (*Rana*). (**E**) A reptile (*Chelone*). (**F**) A bird (*Gallus*). (**G**) A mammal (*Oryctolagus*). (**H**) Another mammal (the cat, *Felis*).

brain and spinal cord form a more less straight tube. In the bipedal condition, which is most developed in man, the eyes are lined up in a plane at right angles to the axis of the spinal column; this necessitates a sharp bend in the axis of the central nervous system. Another source of variation is the importance of the sense of smell (olfaction). Many mammals rely heavily on olfaction for their survival, whereas others are more dependent on their eyes and ears than on their noses. Correspondingly differences in the brain reflect the relative importances of the special senses. Animals in which olfaction predominates are **macrosmatic,** whereas those that rely less on their noses are **microsmatic.** The insectivores

and rodents are macrosmatic mammals; primates and cetaceans (whales, porpoises, dolphins) are microsmatic. Carnivores such as the dog and cat are intermediate. The microsmatic animals are often endowed with high intelligence.

Why Do Tracts Cross the Midline?

Students often ask why it is that so many central pathways include decussations. This chapter is the only one in the book appropriate for a brief discussion of the question.

There is no obvious advantage in having

decussating tracts connecting the brain and spinal cord. All systems dealing with both sides of the body are, in any case, provided with commissural fibers. Indeed, the vestibular system and cerebellum work in conjunction with the ipsilateral sides in a perfectly efficient manner. Even in the visual system, commissural connections might provide for binocular vision if each eye were connected only to the same side of the brain.

The only comprehensible explanations for crossing of tracts are those advanced by comparative neuroanatomists, who cite decussations as an example of the continued exploitation of a structural feature that helped our lowly ancestors to overcome their even more lowly competitors. Natural selection would not allow the loss of a decussating pathway if this were an advantage in a world full of other animals with nondecussating neural connections. In order to have left and right sides, all the competing creatures would have to be bilaterally symmetrical, with different dorsal and ventral surfaces. The struggle for survival is therefore supposed to have been among animals that lived on land or in shallow water, where "dorsal" and "ventral" would have meant something. Even the most primitive nervous systems include motor and sensory neurons. A potentially fatal stimulus can be expected to evoke a movement of withdrawal, so that the individual may survive and reproduce itself. The attacked animal is more likely to escape by moving away from the assaulted side, especially if the predator is not smart enough to predict such a response. The fastest neuronal circuit for stimulating withdrawal to the other side of the midline is a sensory neuron whose axon crosses the midline to contact motor neurons that make their nearest muscle fibers contract. Such an arrangement makes wormlike creatures bend away from the attacked side. It may be significant that even in man the midline is crossed at a more caudal (presumably more primitive) level in the pathway for pain than in the pathway for discriminative sensations (see Chap. 15).

Chapter 13

Peripheral Nerve Endings and Axon Reflexes

Nerve endings are the sites at which the nervous system receives and transmits information. Some endings are neurites; in others the neurites interact with other cells. The simplest response of nervous tissue is an axon reflex, in which signals are received and transmitted by branches of the same neurite.

Receptive Endings

A suitable stimulus applied to a receptor results in a signal being sent along a sensory neurite. With most receptors, the signal is an impulse (action potential) in an axon. Usually the frequency of action potentials in a sensory axon varies proportionally with the intensity of the stimulus.

Repeated stimulation of any receptor causes it to stop sending signals along its nerve fiber. This is called **adaptation.** Some receptors are *rapidly adapting,* so they respond principally to changes. Others are *very slowly adapting,* and therefore respond continuously to the stimuli that activate them. Receptors for cold and warmth provide examples of *moderately slowly adapting* receptors: It is difficult to estimate the exact temperature of an object, but small changes in temperature are easily and quickly recognized.

Cutaneous Sensory Innervation

The skin contains many types of sensory nerve endings. The distal branches of the axons of dorsal root ganglion cells branch profusely beneath and within the skin, and form plexuses in the subcutaneous connective tissue and in the dermis. The most richly innervated areas are those capable of highly discriminative tactile sensation, such as the fingers and the face. The endings of some sensory axons are associated with other cells, which sometimes form a capsule, or with the roots (follicles) of hairs. These endings all detect mechanical stimuli. Other axonal branches end freely, and are variously sensitive to mechanical displacements, to changes in temperature, and to those harmful stimuli that are perceived as pain.

Different types of stimulus excite different endings, but the identifiable types of ending cannot individually be correlated with the kinds of sensation (**modalities**) consciously felt and named by human beings. Knowledge of the structural and functional identities of peripheral sensory nerve endings has come largely from electrophysiological experimentation in animals. Most of the receptors studied in animals have structurally similar counterparts in man. Table 13-1 lists the best understood cutaneous receptors and their

Table 13-1. Sensory Endings in Skin

Name and Location	Structural Features	Function
Free nerve endings (in hairy and hairless skin)	Unmyelinated terminal parts of axons, mostly in superficial zone of dermis. Some enter epidermis	Involved in all types of touch, temperature, and pain. Physiologically different types cannot be recognized morphologically
Merkel* endings (in hairy and hairless skin)	The Merkel* cell in the basal layer of the epidermis contains granules that resemble synaptic vesicles. It is in contact with an expanded axonal ending (tactile meniscus). A *Haarscheibe,* or "touch dome," is a spot in hairy skin containing many Merkel cells supplied by branches of a single axon. *Haarscheiben* are most abundant in furry beasts, but infrequent in man	Slowly adapting touch receptors. They deliver trains of impulses in response to sustained pressure upon the skin
Peritrichial endings (in hairy skin)	Several axons encircle each hair follicle, with terminal branches apposed to the outer root sheath	Rapidly adapting receptors, giving rise to a burst of impulses whenever the hair is moved, but no response during sustained deformation of the hair
Ruffini* endings (in hairy and hairless skin, in subcutaneous connective tissue)	Elongated, encapsulated corpuscle, lying horizontally	Slowly adapting; sustained response to stretching in the plane of the surface of the skin
Pacinian* corpuscles (in hairy and hairless skin, in underlying connective tissue; also in connective tissues elsewhere)	Ellipsoidal, with a capsule of many layers of cells and a single central axon (also called Vater–Pacini* corpuscles)	Very rapidly adapting response to deformation. Detects vibration in skin and other tissues
Meissner's* corpuscles (in dermis of papillary ridges of hairless skin, especially tips of fingers)	Several axons have terminal branches in a cellular capsule whose long axis is perpendicular to the epidermal surface	Rapidly adapting response to gentle friction of surface of skin, for the discrimination of textures of surfaces of objects
End-bulbs (in dermis of hairless skin around eyes, mouth, anus, genital and urinary orifices)	Spheroidal, encapsulated endings. Several named variants in mammals and birds	Functions uncertain, but probably respond to mechanical stimuli

Eponyms: G. Meissner (1829–1905)—German anatomist; also described submucous plexus (see Chap. 27). F.S. Merkel (1845–1919)—German anatomist. F. Pacini (1812–1883)—Italian histologist. A. Ruffini (1864–1928)—Another Italian histologist. A. Vater (1684–1751)—Another German anatomist.

functions. Some are illustrated in Figure 13-1.

The encapsulated tactile endings (Meissner's, Pacini's, Ruffini's) are connected with rapidly conducting (group Aβ: Ib and II) nerve fibers. Peritrichial endings and free nerve endings subserving touch are branches of myelinated fibers with a wider range of conduction velocities (groups Aβ and Aδ). Unmyelinated (group C) sensory axons termi-

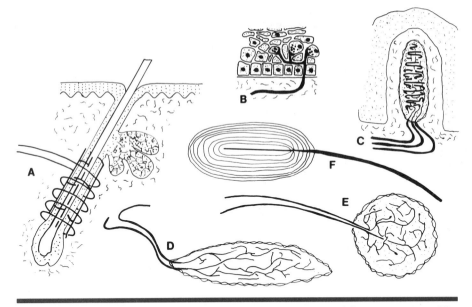

Figure 13-1   Sensory nerve-endings in skin. (A) Peritrichial endings. **(B)** Merkel endings. **(C)** Meissner's corpuscle. **(D)** Ruffini ending. **(E)** An end-bulb. **(F)** Pacinian corpuscle. (For more information, see Table 13-1.)

nate only as free nerve endings (see Table 2-2 for fiber-types in peripheral nerves). The perception of pain and temperature is a function of the Aδ and C fibers.

Proprioceptive End-Organs

Important information about position and movement of parts of the body comes from cutaneous and similar, more deeply placed receptors, which respond to pressure. Exclusively proprioceptive end-organs are located in muscles and tendons and in the capsules and ligaments of joints. Conscious awareness of position and movement comes principally from the proprioceptive organs of muscles. Proprioceptive information that never impinges on consciousness is also generated by the sensory endings in muscles, as well as by those in tendons and in the joints themselves.

The **neuromuscular spindle** is the most complicated of the sensory end-organs described

in this chapter. It is important to know how the spindle works, because its activities are essential for all useful movement. The account given here is greatly simplified.

Each neuromuscular spindle (Fig. 13-2) consists of a few modified muscle fibers contained in a collagenous capsule. The capsule is joined at both ends to connective tissue that is continuous with the tendons or other bony attachments of the muscle. The muscle fibers in the spindle are called **intrafusal fibers.** They differ from the ordinary (**extrafusal**) fibers of the muscle in having the nuclei in the middle and the contractile myofibrils at both ends. An extrafusal fiber has myofibrils and nuclei along its whole length. Whereas the extrafusal muscle fibers are innervated by motor neurons with rapidly conducting axons (Aα), the intrafusal fibers are supplied by small neurons with thinner axons (Aγ). The two types of motor neuron are commonly called alpha and gamma-efferent neurons.

The intrafusal fibers are contacted by sen-

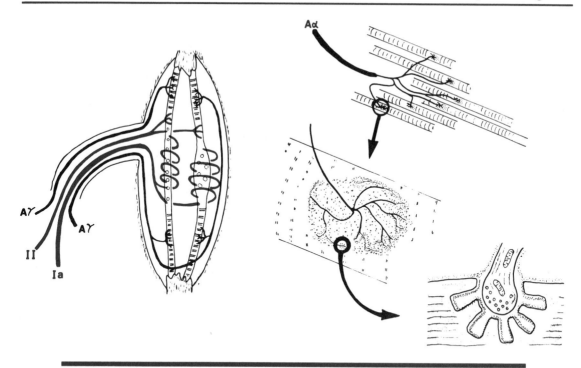

Figure 13-2 Nerve-endings in muscle. (*Left*) A neuromuscular spindle with sensory (colored) and motor innervation. (*Right*) Motor end-plate at successively higher magnifications. The colored stippling indicates the distribution of acetylcholinesterase (see Table 3-1) on the postsynaptic surface.

sory, as well as motor, axons. The sensory terminals are applied to the central, noncontractile parts of the intrafusal fiber. They initiate trains of impulses when the middle part of the intrafusal fiber is stretched. Stretching may be due to (a) passive extension of the whole muscle, which pulls on both ends of the spindle, or (b) contraction of the myofibrils of the intrafusal fiber, causing lengthening of the central sensory region.

Two types of sensory ending are present in each spindle. The annulospiral endings, which are terminal branches of group Ia nerve fibers, are rapidly adapting. They therefore respond to the *rate of stretching,* a "phasic" response. The flower-spray endings are from group II fibers. They adapt slowly so that they respond to the maintained amount of stretch, thereby signalling the *length of the muscle,* a "tonic" response.

The *tension* in a muscle is monitored by the **neurotendinous spindles** or **Golgi tendon organs,*** supplied by group Ib nerve fibers. The

* Camillo Golgi (1843–1926) was the Italian histologist who described the cytoplasmic organelle that bears his name, and also several cell-types in the nervous system. He developed a staining method that shows occasional neurons with all their neurites. This technique enabled Santiago Felipe Ramon Y Cajal (1852–1934) to provide much evidence in support of the "neuron theory," which maintained that neurons were not in cytoplasmic continuity at synapses. This theory had been proposed by two Swiss scientists: The great embryologist, Wilhelm His (1831–1904), and a clinical neurologist and neuroanatomist, Auguste Henri Forel (1848–1931). Another champion of the theory was the German anatomist Heinrich Wilhelm Gottfried Waldeyer-Hartz (1836–1921). Golgi himself preferred the alternative hypothesis of cytoplasmic continuity between nerve cells. Ramon y Cajal, a Spaniard, contributed more to neurohistology than profuse terminal branches of the axons end among collagen fibers in encapsulated regions within the tendon.

The ligaments and capsules of joints contain encapsulated nerve endings similar to some of those in skin. These receptors respond to positions and movements of joints, but their input to the central nervous system is probably involved only in the unconscious (reflex) control of movements. The muscle spindles are the receptors principally responsible for conscious awareness of position and movements of joints. There are also many free nerve endings in and around joints, and these give rise to the severe pain that is felt whenever a joint is injured or inflamed. These pain-sensitive endings have central connections in the spinal cord that provoke contraction of the muscles acting upon the painful joint, providing limitation of movement and protection against further injury.

Visceral Receptors

Some of the sensory nerve endings in internal organs are Group C fibers, which evoke **pain** when they are stimulated by excessive stretching or by a deficiency of oxygen. Others are arrays of axonal terminals of special neurons involved in the **regulation of function.** Within the brain there are neurons sensitive to temperature and to various chemical stimuli (see Chaps. 26, 27).

Special Senses

Chemoreceptive cells are involved in smell and taste. Vision involves light-sensitive cells

of the central nervous system. The receptors in the auditory and vestibular systems are epithelial cells that respond to movements in the surrounding liquids. Other chapters are devoted to these special senses.

Effector Endings

The efferent axons of the peripheral nervous system impinge upon skeletal striated muscle fibers, smooth muscle cells, and secretory cells.

The Motor End-Plate

The contact between a terminal branch of the axon of a motor neuron and a striated muscle fiber is illustrated in Figure 13-2. The neuromuscular junction resembles a typical synapse, differing mainly in the wider synaptic cleft and the greatly folded postsynaptic membrane. The transmitter is **acetylcholine (ACh)** which, if released in sufficient amount, depolarizes the muscle cell membrane and triggers contraction. Small, transient reductions in the resting membrane potential can be recorded by microelectrodes in muscle fibers that are not contracting. These miniature end-plate potentials (**MEPPs**) are due to the leakage of small amounts of ACh, possibly from individual synaptic vesicles. The arrival of an impulse causes a large number of MEPPs to summate, because of the much larger amount of transmitter that is then released into the synaptic cleft. **Acetylcholinesterase,** the enzyme that catalyzes the hydrolysis of ACh, is present in the basal lamina of the postsynaptic membrane.

The **acetylcholine receptor** molecules are normally confined to the postsynaptic region of the surface of the muscle fiber. This restriction is caused by the presence of the presynaptic bouton. If a muscle is denervated by

---

any other investigator. He prepared detailed descriptions of the nervous systems of man and other animals and made important studies of axonal degeneration and regeneration. In 1906 he and Golgi shared the Nobel prize for Physiology or Medicine.

cutting its motor nerve, its cells synthesize larger numbers of acetylcholine receptors and insert them into all parts of the cell membrane. The muscle cells then become responsive to unphysiologically low concentrations of ACh. This is called *denervation supersensitivity.*

Myasthenia gravis is an autoimmune disease in which antibodies inactivate the acetylcholine receptors of skeletal muscles, thereby interfering with neuromuscular synaptic transmission. The resulting weakness (total paralysis in severe cases) can be ameliorated by drugs such as **eserine, neostigmine** and several organophosphorus compounds that inhibit acetylcholinesterase, making more ACh available to the receptors spared by the disease.

The same **anticholinesterases** are used to reverse the paralyzing actions of **tubocurarine** (a curare alkaloid) and **gallamine,** drugs that competitively inhibit the combination of ACh with its receptors in the motor end-plate. Tubocurarine and gallamine are valuable in surgery because they inhibit spontaneous respiratory movements. A similar drug with much briefer action is **suxamethonium,** which acts for only 2 minutes. The transient paralysis of the vocal cords makes it easy for an anesthetist to insert a tube into his patient's trachea.

Autonomic Axonal Terminals

The axons of the neurons of autonomic ganglia are unmyelinated. They branch profusely in the organs they supply. Their terminal parts have many swellings, known as **varicosities,** with the ultrastructural features of boutons terminaux. The neurotransmitters (notably acetylcholine and noradrenaline) are stored in the varicosities and are released from them by action potentials. Postsynaptic specializations are not usually evident. Usually the transmitter has to diffuse through the extracellular fluid for several μm before reaching the cells upon which it acts.

Axon Reflexes

The Triple Response

A minor injury to the skin, such as a scratch or a hard rub, causes pain and evokes a reaction from the nearby blood vessels. The reaction has three components. At first a *red line* appears at the exact site of injury; it is due to dilatation of capillary vessels. After a few minutes, a swelling in the dermis, called a *wheal,* replaces the red line: The swelling is due to exudation of plasma from capillaries and small venules in the injured skin. The red line and the wheal are produced by **mediators,** which are released from injured cells. The best known is **histamine.** This is one of several mediators secreted by **mast cells,** which occur abundantly in the dermal connective tissue. Before the wheal is fully developed, small arteries dilate in the area surrounding the injury, producing a *flare* of warm, pink skin. Vascular permeability is slightly increased in the region of the flare, but not as much as at the exact site of injury.

The red line, flare, and wheal constitute the **triple response,** which is associated with the name of Thomas Lewis (1881–1945). He was an English physician who contributed importantly to the experimental study of human physiology. The response, which occurs in the skin and some mucous membranes, has also been investigated in laboratory mammals and amphibians.

An injury to skin that has been denervated for more than about a week evokes the red line and wheal, but not the flare. A flare alone develops if the distal stump of a cut cutaneous nerve or dorsal spinal root is electrically stimulated. These and other observations indicate that the flare is mediated by an **axon reflex;** a

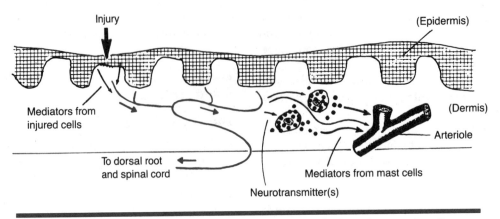

Figure 13-3 Mediation of axon reflex vasodilatation in injured skin. Colored arrows show directions of propagation of nerve impulses. Black arrows show movements of chemical mediators through the extracellular space of the dermis.

neural response that does not involve any synapses. The impulses involved in axon reflex vasodilatation are carried only in certain unmyelinated sensory fibers that contain **substance P,** a peptide neurotransmitter. The reflex is initiated by mediators that act upon the axonal terminals. Impulses travel into other branches of the same axon, which release substance P. The released substance P causes dilatation of small arteries and causes mast cells to secrete their mediators, which also contribute to the vasodilatation.

Neurogenic Inflammation

Many irritant chemicals cause pain, redness, and swelling if they are applied to the skin. Both the vasodilatation and the vascular permeability are much less in denervated than in normal skin. The inflammation and pain are prevented by prior administration of **cap-saicin** in doses that cause degeneration of those nerve fibers that contain substance P. Capsaicin, the pungent principle of red pepper, is itself an irritant, but is unusual in that repeated local applications (or systemic administration, in animals) cause degeneration of the axons whose terminals are stimulated. Thus, the substance P-containing pain-sensitive axons are necessary for production of inflammation by chemical irritants. As with the axon reflex flare, mediators from mast cells are also involved in neurogenic inflammation (Fig. 13-3).

Vasodilatation in the area of skin supplied by an electrically stimulated peripheral nerve or dorsal root is a result of release of substance P and mast cell-derived mediators. Observation of such **antidromic vasodilatation** has been used to provide anatomical evidence of the extent of dermatomes in man, especially by Otfrid Foerster (1873–1941), a German neurosurgeon.

Chapter 14

The Olfactory System

Olfaction is the sensory detection of gases and of finely dispersed liquids (aerosols) that enter the nose. The olfactory system consists of the sensory region of the nasal epithelium, the olfactory nerves, and various parts of the telencephalon. The parts of the brain with anatomically obvious olfactory function are sometimes named the **rhinencephalon** (from the Greek for "nose" and "brain"), but this term has also been applied to many other parts of the forebrain that are only indirectly connected with the olfactory system. It is therefore preferable to avoid the use of "rhinencephalon."

Olfactory Epithelium and Nerves

The **olfactory epithelium** covers the roof of the nasal cavity and the upper parts of the lateral and medial walls. It is pseudostratified, as is the ordinary respiratory epithelium of the nose, but is much thicker. A pseudostratified epithelium is only one layer of cells thick, but looks thicker because the cells are tall and thin. Three types of cells are present in the olfactory epithelium (Fig. 14-1). The connective tissue underlying the epithelium contains bundles of olfactory nerve fibers, blood vessels, and the olfactory glands of Bowman.*

---

* William Bowman (1816–1892) was an English anatomist who also practiced ophthalmology. The capsule of the renal glomerulus and a layer of the cornea also are named after him.

These glands secrete a fluid that covers the surface of the olfactory epithelium. To be smelled, a substance must dissolve in this film of fluid.

The **olfactory neurosensory cells** are bipolar neurons. Each has a dendrite with an expanded end from which cilia project into the layer of secretion on the epithelial surface. Receptor molecules on the cilia combine with odorous substances and cause reduction of the membrane potential. An adequate stimulus depolarizes the surface membrane of the neuron and initiates an action potential (that is, a nerve impulse). The axon of an olfactory neurosensory cell emerges at the basal pole, pierces the basal lamina of the epithelium, and enters the underlying connective tissue.

The olfactory neurosensory cells are the only neurons of vertebrate animals that occur in an epithelium, physiologically at the external surface of the body. They are easily killed, especially by infection or by chemical irritants. Dead neurons are replaced by mitosis and subsequent differentiation of the basal cells. This is the only known instance of replacement of neurons. In the mouse, each olfactory neurosensory cell has a life span of about 40 days, but the cells live much longer in animals carefully protected from nasal infections. Probably the olfactory neurons are replaced to compensate for losses due to wear and tear rather than as part of a regular cyclic turnover.

It is a point of great interest to neurobiologists that whenever a new olfactory neuron

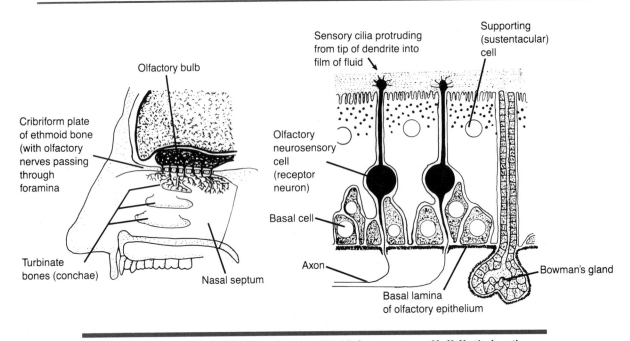

Figure 14-1 The olfactory epithelium and nerves. (*Right*) Gross anatomy. (*Left*) Vertical section through the olfactory epithelium showing features resolved by electron microscopy.

is generated its axon grows through an olfactory nerve and into the olfactory bulb, which is part of the central nervous system. Comparable axonal growth from the peripheral into the central nervous system cannot occur in spinal nerves. If a dorsal root is crushed between the ganglion and the spinal cord, axons regenerate only as far as the junction of peripheral with central neuroglial cells.

The unmyelinated axons of the olfactory neurosensory cells are the thinnest anywhere, being only 0.1 to 0.5 μm in diameter. Several are ensheathed in a single mesaxon of a neurolemmal cell. The little bundles of olfactory axons join together to form about 20 **olfactory nerves** on each side of the midline. The nerves pass through foramina in the cribriform plate of the ethmoid bone, which separates the nasal cavity from the cranial cavity. Within the cranium, the olfactory nerves pierce the dura and are ensheathed by the arachnoid and pia before entering the **olfactory bulb.**

Anosmia

Loss of the sense of smell is most often due to the common cold, in which odorous substances are kept away from the olfactory epithelium by excessive mucus in the nose. A head injury may fracture the cribriform plate and sever the olfactory nerves. The result is **anosmia** (loss of sense of smell), which may be bilateral or unilateral, depending on the extent of the damage. In testing smell, it is important not to use irritant or pungent substances which stimulate non-olfactory nerve endings in the nose.

Another consequence of injury to the cribriform plate is **cerebrospinal fluid rhinorrhea:** colorless liquid runs from the nose because the subarachnoid space around the brain has been put in continuity with the nasal cavity. This condition is associated with the risk of infection spreading from the nose into the cerebrospinal fluid, causing meningitis.

Central Olfactory Pathways

In the **olfactory bulb,** the axons from the olfactory nerves end in synaptic complexes called glomeruli. The postsynaptic neurites in an olfactory glomerulus are the dendrites of **mitral cells,** which are the principal cells of the olfactory bulb. These synapses are excitatory; the transmitter may be carnosine. The olfactory bulb also contains two types of interneurons, both inhibitory to the mitral cells. The periglomerular cells are GABAergic, and the granule cells (whose only processes are dendrites) are dopaminergic. Both types of inhibitory interneurons receive afferent fibers from parts of the brain caudal to the olfactory bulb.

The axons of the mitral cells, together with fibers projecting rostrally to the bulb, constitute the **olfactory tract,** which lies on the ventral (inferior) surface of the frontal lobe. The olfactory tract ends at the rostral (anterior) border of the **anterior perforated substance,** which is an area pierced by many small arteries anterior to the optic tract and lateral to the chiasma (Fig. 14-2). Most mitral cell axons turn laterally as the **lateral olfactory stria** and continue to their sites of termination in the cortex of the **uncus** and **limen insulae,** and in the **corticomedial nuclei of the amygdala.** Smaller numbers of fibers of the olfactory tract form the **intermediate olfactory stria.** They end in certain nuclei within the **anterior perforated substance.** In gross anatomy, a ridge called the

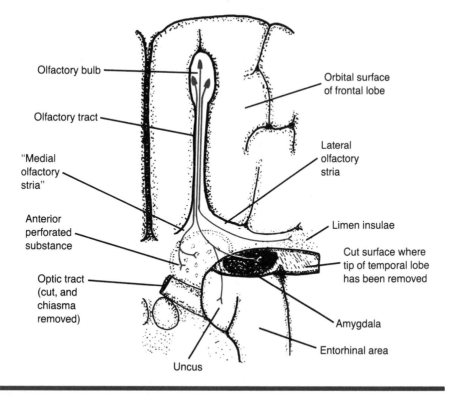

Figure 14-2 Central olfactory pathways (colored) projected onto the ventral surface of the left cerebral hemisphere. The tip of the temporal lobe has been cut off. (The ridge named "medial olfactory stria" does not contain fibers from the olfactory bulb.)

"medial olfactory stria" also is recognized. Once it was thought that fibers from the olfactory tract went through the medial olfactory stria to the septal area. Now it is known that this connection does not exist, and that the medial olfactory stria is not a real tract at all.

The sites of termination of the olfactory tract are all cortical areas. They are connected by association fibers with other regions of the cerebral cortex, notably the entorhinal area at the rostral (anterior) end of the parahippocampal gyrus, and the cortex of the ventral (inferior, or orbital) surface of the frontal lobe, lateral to the olfactory tract. The latter cortical areas are **association cortex** for olfaction. Their integrity is necessary for the conscious identification of different odors and for responses of the autonomic nervous system to certain smells. For example, the smell of food provokes salivation and secretion of gastric juice. Other smells cause nausea, or even vomiting, with a sense of revulsion that encourages withdrawal from a possibly poisonous substance.

Although no thalamic nucleus intervenes between the olfactory epithelium and the cerebral cortex, there are extensive connections between the frontal lobe and the mediodorsal nucleus of the thalamus. This thalamic nucleus is also connected with the hypothalamus, providing a pathway to the nuclei in the brain stem and the spinal cord that send preganglionic fibers to the ganglia of the autonomic nervous system. The connections of the limbic system, which includes the entorhinal area, provide pathways connecting the olfactory system with many parts of the brain, including those associated with autonomic function.

The axons of some mitral cells end in the **anterior olfactory nucleus,** which consists of groups of neurons in the olfactory tract, mostly at its rostral and caudal ends. The axons of some neurons in the anterior olfactory nucleus project back to the olfactory bulb.

Other neurons of the nucleus send their axons across the midline in the anterior commissure, and then along the contralateral olfactory tract to the bulb. There are other efferent fibers in the olfactory tract, too; most of the them arise from neurons in and near the anterior perforated substance. All axons that project rostrally to the bulb end by synapsing with the interneurons there. Together with the internal neuronal circuitry of the bulb, the efferent fibers of the olfactory tract are involved in the processing of olfactory information. One function of these connections is to facilitate paying attention to significant odors and ignoring smells that are everywhere and do not need to be noticed.

In conscious experience, the sense of smell is closely associated with that of taste. The central pathways for these two chemical senses, however, are surprisingly separate from one another. One point of overlap may be the cortex of the insula, where thalamocortical fibers of the taste pathway end no great distance from the termination sites of some of the fibers of the lateral olfactory stria. The name "limen insulae" means "threshold of the island"—an insect crawling into the lateral sulcus from the ventral (inferior) surface of the cerebrum would have to pass over the limen before it could mount the gyri of the insula.

Olfactory Hallucinations

The temporal lobe is a common site of origin of uncontrolled bursts of excitatory neuronal impulses, or epilepsy (see Chap. 22). One of the first events in a seizure of this kind is often the awareness of an unpleasant, unnatural odor. Such as episode is called an **uncinate attack,** because the sensation is attributed to abnormal activity of neurons in the uncus.

Uncal Herniation

Pressure on the cerebral hemispheres by a rapidly enlarging lesion, such as a hemorrhage into the space between the dura and the arachnoid, causes the midbrain, the diencephalon, and the uncus to be forced down into the notch in the tentorium cerebelli. The first sign of this occurrence is dysfunction of the preganglionic parasympathetic fibers in the oculomotor nerve, and this is followed by damage to the midbrain itself. In fatal cases, a groove in the rostral (anterior) end of the parahippocampal gyrus of each side shows where the unci too have been forced into the tentorial notch. Uncinate attacks sometimes occur in patients who recover from tentorial herniation.

The Vomeronasal System

This system is absent in man, but is of such great importance to almost all other mammals that it is mentioned briefly here. The *vomer* (Latin for ploughshare) is one of the bones of the nasal septum. At the rostral end of each surface of the septum, just dorsal to the hard palate, there is a narrow, blind-ended tunnel in the bone, communicating rostrally with the nasal cavity. This tunnel contains the **vomeronasal organ.** The organ is a tube lined by sensory epithelium similar to the olfactory epithelium. The connective tissue between this epithelium and the bony wall of the tunnel contains blood vessels, which are innervated by noradrenergic axons from the superior cervical sympathetic ganglion.

The axons of the neurosensory cells of the vomeronasal organ form the **vomeronasal nerve,** which passes through the cribriform plate and ends in the accessory olfactory bulb, a group of neurons lateral to the main olfactory bulb.

The orifice of the vomeronasal organ is directly above the **nasopalatine foramen,** a small hole, through which the nasal and oral cavities communicate, behind the incisor tooth. Chemical agents that stimulate the vomeronasal receptors are deposited as liquid droplets near the orifice of the organ, either by the tongue or by sniffing into the nose. Sympathetic innervation then causes constriction of the vomeronasal blood vessels so that the central cavity of the organ is enlarged. Any liquid near the orifice is thereby sucked in and brought into contact with the cilia of the neurosensory cells.

The vomeronasal system is used for the identification of chemical agents (**pheromones**) secreted or excreted by other individuals of the same species. Chemical stimuli that act upon the vomeronasal organ include sex-attractant substances and materials deposited for the purposes of marking territory. Animals with obstructed vomeronasal organs fail to recognize such chemical signals. The vomeronasal organ is not involved in chemical sensation associated with feeding, which is a function of the olfactory and gustatory systems. The ordinary olfactory system, which detects gases rather than liquids, is not used for the detection of pheromones emitted by potential mates or rivals.

Chapter 15

Somatic Sensation

The exteroceptive pathways are concerned with sensation from the skin, mucous membranes, subcutaneous connective tissue, and deeper structures such as muscles and bones, which can perceive pressure applied through the skin. The interoceptive pathways transmit conscious proprioception (also called kinesthesia), which is awareness of position and movement. The **somesthetic pathways** are the arrangements of neurons that conduct somatic sensory information to the cerebral cortex. A great deal of proprioceptive neural signalling does not give rise to conscious sensation, but is concerned with spinal reflexes and the activity of the cerebellum. These unconscious pathways are not considered in this chapter. Activity of somatic afferent neurons also contributes to the state of consciousness itself, through pathways involving the reticular formation of the brain stem.

Modalities of Sensation

By physiological experimentation it is possible to identify a variety of types of physical stimulus, each giving rise to characteristic activity in individual axons of nerves. Several kinds of mechanical stimulus can be associated with histologically identifiable receptor organs. For other sensations, such as warmth, cold, and simple touching of the skin, specific sensory end-organs cannot be recognized under the microscope. The receptors are therefore presumed to be terminal axonal branches of nondescript appearance. A **modality** is a type of sensation that can be simply described in ordinary language, such as "warmth," "pressure," or "itch." It may be due to impulses in more than one kind of afferent neuron. *Certain modalities are valuable in descriptive neuroanatomy and in diagnostic clinical neurology because they give rise to activity in different ascending pathways.*

Discrimination and Cognition

For some cutaneous modalities, including pain and changes of temperature, precise spatial localization of the stimulus is not possible. For others, notably touch, the stimulus can be exactly localized, and it is possible to resolve points of simultaneous contact that are close together (two-point discrimination). Accurate knowledge is also gained about shapes and about the changing direction and position of an object moving while in contact with the skin. The latter sensibilities are needed for the identification of solid objects (stereognosis) by touching and feeling. The degree of resolution or discrimination reflects the richness of the innervation of the skin by axons responding to various kinds of stimulus. Similar considerations apply also to deeper structures. Thus the position and movements of a joint can normally be described with great accuracy. However, the localization of pain from diseased joints, muscles, or teeth is crude and quite often inaccurate.

A person's correct identification of a sensory stimulus requires not only the integrity of the peripheral innervation and the appropriate somesthetic pathway, but also the proper functioning of the cerebral cortex. The cortex is the site of interpretation of the sensory signals, and it is also responsible for producing the words used to describe them. It may not always be easy to determine whether apparently defective sensation is due to damage in an ascending pathway or in the cerebral cortex. (For disorders of cognition due to cortical lesions, see Chap. 22.)

General Features of the Long Ascending Pathways

A somesthetic pathway is traced from the periphery (skin, muscle, joint) to the **first somatosensory area** of the cerebral cortex, which occupies the **postcentral gyrus.** Throughout a pathway, each part of the body is represented by a group of neurons or axons in a particular position. Such spatial representation in the central nervous system is called **somatotopic representation** (from Greek words for "body" and "place"). In the first somatosensory area, the contralateral half of the body forms an upside-down pattern, with the foot and perineum on the medial surface of the hemisphere, and the head above the lateral sulcus. Somatic sensations are consciously appreciated as the result of neural interaction between the first somatosensory area and the nearby association cortex of the parietal lobe.

Each pathway is a series of at least three populations of neurons. The first in the series are unipolar neurons of sensory ganglia. The synapses in a pathway are not merely relays, which would be unnecessary, but they allow for **convergence,** so that a large region of the body is represented in progressively smaller regions of the central nervous system. The synapses also permit modification of the ascending signals by other sensory inputs and by descending tracts. One effect of inhibition by descending pathways is protection of the cerebral cortex from "noise," or unwanted sensory information.

Sensory signals from one side of the body are sent to the cerebral hemisphere of the other side. In each pathway, neurons with somata in either the spinal cord or the brain stem have axons that cross the midline on their way to the contralateral thalamus. The final link in every somesthetic pathway is a thalamocortical projection.

The Spinothalamic System

This is also called the "anterolateral pathway," from the position of the spinothalamic tract in the spinal cord. It deals with the modalities of **pain, temperature,** and **touch,** excluding the finer discriminative tactile abilities. The pathway to the somatosensory cortex consists of three populations of neurons. The positions of their somata and axons are shown by the thick lines in Figure 15-1.

The following features of the spinothalamic system are particularly important:

1. The central branch of the axon of the first order neuron ends in the dorsal horn of the spinal gray matter.
2. The axon of the second order neuron crosses the midline in the spinal cord, usually about one segment rostral to the nerve root with which it is concerned.
3. The crossing fibers are in the white matter immediately ventral to the central canal of the spinal cord.
4. The spinothalamic tract (spinal lemniscus) is laterally placed in the medulla, pons, and midbrain (see Chap. 8).
5. The spinothalamic system converges with the medial lemniscus system (described below) in the ventral posterior lateral (VPL) nucleus of the thalamus. The thal-

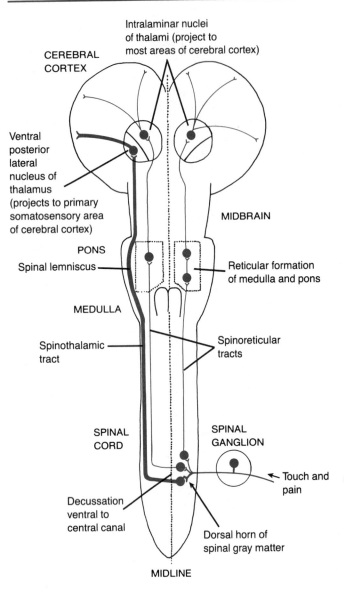

Intralaminar nuclei
of thalami (project to
most areas of cerebral cortex)

CEREBRAL
CORTEX

Ventral
posterior
lateral
nucleus of
thalamus
(projects to primary
somatosensory area
of cerebral cortex)

MIDBRAIN

PONS

Spinal lemniscus

Reticular formation
of medulla and pons

MEDULLA

Spinothalamic
tract

Spinoreticular
tracts

SPINAL
CORD

SPINAL
GANGLION

Touch and
pain

Decussation
ventral to
central canal

Dorsal horn of
spinal gray matter

MIDLINE

Figure 15-1   The spinothalamic system. The thick lines show the pathways for sensations (notably of touch, warmth, and coldness) that can be accurately localized. Thinner lines show pathways for poorly localized components of sensation, especially pain. (For positions of tracts, see figures in Chap. 7 and 8.)

amocortical projections are therefore the same for both systems.

The spinothalamic system is not as simple as might be inferred from this brief account. There are connections involving interneurons in the dorsal horn (mentioned below in connection with pain), and connections with the reticular formation, the periaqueductal gray and thalamic nuclei other than the VPL.

Pain

A tissue becomes painful when some of the cells in it are severely deformed or killed as a result, for example, of mechanical trauma, extremes of temperature, inadequate oxygen supply (ischemia), or stretching and swelling due to inflammatory or neoplastic disease. Substances known as **mediators** are released from damaged cells. Known mediators include potassium ions, prostaglandins of the "E" series, histamine, and proteolytic enzymes. These substances initiate trains of impulses in fine myelinated (group Aδ) and unmyelinated (group C) axons. They also make small blood vessels dilate and become permeable to proteins in the plasma of the blood. The resulting pain, vasodilatation, and swelling constitute **inflammation** of the tissue.

The unipolar cell bodies of the A and C axons (collectively called **nociceptive fibers**) are in the dorsal root ganglion. The central branches of their axons end in the **dorsal horn.** There they synapse with neurons (in laminae I and V) that give rise to the **spinothalamic and spinoreticular tracts,** and also with interneurons (in lamina II, the substantia gelatinosa). The dorsal horn also receives thicker myelinated axons (group A) concerned with modalities other than pain. The circuitry is shown in Figure 7-3. (For the head, equivalent connections exist in the caudal part of the spinal trigeminal nucleus.) According to the **gate theory** of pain, this circuitry compares the nociceptive with the non-nociceptive input. If the former predominates, impulses reporting pain are sent up the spinothalamic and spinoreticular tracts. It is sometimes possible to suppress the perception of pain by presenting the dorsal horn with additional sensory signals. This can be done by rubbing, warming, or cooling the skin, or by making it feel warm with a mildly irritant liniment. Suppression of pain can also be obtained by applying low voltage electrical pulses to nerves; such pulses stimulate the larger group A fibers, but not the small nociceptive ones. Competition among different afferent inputs may be partially involved in relief of pain by the oriental practice of acupuncture. This involves sticking needles in the skin, but commonly into an area innervated by a segmental nerve different from that supplying the source of the pain.

The upward transmission of signals for pain is principally through the spinothalamic system to be contralateral thalamus and somatosensory cortex. However, *there is also appreciable transmission bilaterally* through spinoreticular and reticulothalamic pathways, and thence to extensive areas of the cerebral cortex (thin lines in Fig. 15-1).

Attempts to relieve intractable pain surgically by cutting through the ventrolateral spinal white matter are often unsuccessful; the ability to localize the pain is lost, but the sensation persists and may even get worse with time. It is probable that other ascending pathways take over the function of the transected tracts. Lesions in the thalamus can cause ordinarily harmless stimuli to be felt as severe pain; the neurophysiological basis of this condition, the **thalamic syndrome,** is not understood.

Medial Lemniscus System

This pathway is also called the "dorsal (or posterior) column system," because it includes axons ascending in the gracile and cuneate fasciculi of the spinal cord. It is concerned with *discriminative sensations,* both tactile and proprioceptive. The integrity of the medial lemniscus system is necessary for all discriminative tactile sensation and for proprioception in the upper limb. (*Proprioception for the lower limb follows a different pathway, described in the next section of this chapter.*)

The sense of vibration, once thought to travel specifically in the gracile and cuneate fasciculi, is now known to be carried in the

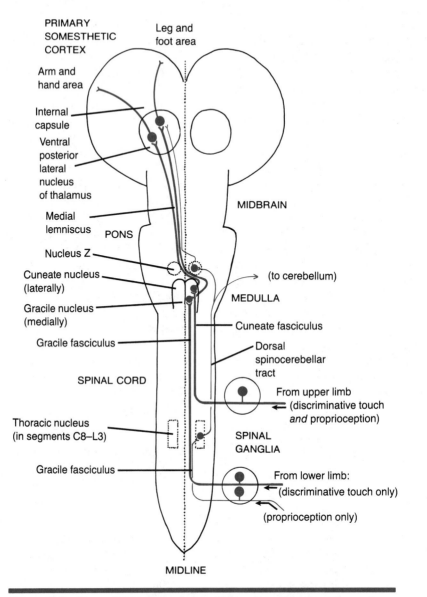

Figure 15-2 The medial lemniscus system. Thicker lines show the pathways for discriminative touch (all levels) and proprioception (upper limb only). Thinner lines show the different pathways for proprioception from the lower limb.

lateral and ventral spinal white matter too. Testing vibration sense is valuable in the examination of suspected diseases of peripheral nerves, but it is of little value in the evaluation of sensory disorders due to lesions of the spinal cord or brain stem.

The following features of the medial lemniscus system (thick lines in Fig. 15-2) are particularly important:

1. The axon of the primary sensory neuron has two long branches. One goes to the

periphery, and the other ascends to the gracile or cuneate nucleus in the medulla.

2. The system is entirely ipsilateral in the spinal cord.

3. The gracile fasciculus and nucleus are concerned with the lower spinal segments, and the cuneate fasciculus and nucleus with the upper segments. Consequently, the cuneate fasciculus is not present below the midthoracic level of the cord.

4. The second order neurons, in the gracile and cuneate nuclei, give rise to axons that cross the midline in the closed part of the medulla and then ascend through the brain stem as the medial lemniscus.

5. The medial lemniscus is near the midline in the medulla. It occupies a progressively more lateral position as it ascends through the pons and midbrain (see Chap. 8), but it is always medial to the spinal lemniscus.

6. The thalamocortical connection is the same as that for the spinothalamic system.

The medial lemniscus system also includes some axons that originate from somata in the dorsal horn. Some of these ascend in the gracile and cuneate fasciculi, others in the dorsal part of the lateral white matter of the cord. These fibers are not shown in Figure 15-2.

Proprioception From the Upper and Lower Limbs

The pathways for conscious proprioception are also shown in Figure 15-2. For the upper limb, the pathway is identical to that for discriminative tactile sensation. For the lower limb (thin lines in Fig. 15-2), the central branches of the axons of the first order neurons ascend in the gracile fasciculus only as far as the thoracic nucleus (Clarke's column) in segments C8 to L3, where they terminate. The neurons in Clarke's column give rise to

the dorsal spinocerebellar tract. The axons of the tract have branches in the medulla that go to nucleus Z (of Brodal and Pompeiano), a group of cells rostral to the gracile nucleus. Nucleus Z contributes internal arcuate fibers that enter the contralateral medial lemniscus.*

Thus, *the proprioceptive pathway for the lower limb is distinctive* in that: (a) It is a chain of four (rather than three) populations of neurons; and (b) in the upper spinal cord the pathway is located in the lateral, not the dorsal, white matter. Proprioception from the lower limbs is therefore not affected by destructive lesions in the gracile funiculus at cervical levels, although tactile sensation is impaired. A lesion in the gracile fasciculus of the upper lumbar cord, on the other hand, causes loss of both conscious proprioception and discriminative tactile sensation in the lower limb.

Spino-cervico-thalamic Pathway

This is an ascending pathway concerned with several sensory modalities in some animals, including the cat and the monkey. Neurons in the dorsal horn project ipsilaterally to the lateral cervical nucleus in segments C1 and C2. This nucleus, which is lateral to the tip of the dorsal horn, gives rise to axons that join the contralateral medial lemniscus. In human spinal cords, the lateral cervical nucleus is either absent or small and inconspicuous. The existence of a spino-cervico-thalamic pathway in man is therefore questionable.

Somatic Sensation from the Head

The **sensory trigeminal nuclei** receive primary afferent axons concerned with somatic sen-

---

Eponyms: Alf Brodal (born 1910) is a Norwegian neuroanatomist. Ottavio Pompeiano (born 1927) is an Italian physiologist. For Clarke, see Chapter 7.

sation in the head. Most of these axons arise from neurons in the trigeminal ganglion; smaller numbers come from the sensory ganglia of the facial, glossopharyngeal, and vagus nerves. The peripheral distributions and central connections of these cranial nerves and the different functions of the trigeminal nuclei are described in Chapter 20.

Second order neurons in the pontine and spinal trigeminal nuclei give rise to axons that cross the midline in the pons and medulla and ascend as the **trigeminal lemniscus** (see Chap. 8). This tract ends in the **ventral posterior medial** (VPM) nucleus of the thalamus. The thalamic neurons project to the head area of the somatosensory cortex, in the postcentral gyrus.

Descending Pathways That Influence Sensation

The proper interpretation of the outside world and the state of the body itself would be impossible if every impulse in every sensory axon were to be brought eventually to the cerebral cortex. An editing system is necessary, so that the cortex can select the sensory information worthy of conscious attention while leaving more humble duties to the spinal cord, brain stem, and cerebellum. The editing function is carried out by descending fibers that terminate in the sites of origin of the ascending tracts. Some of these descending pathways are shown in Figure 15-3.

Descending tracts modify activity in the ascending systems at three levels:

1. In the **dorsal horn** of the spinal gray matter. This is the site of termination of large numbers of corticospinal fibers, mostly from the postcentral gyrus. Other axons ending in the dorsal horn come from the reticular formation and from the gracile and cuneate nuclei. One of the reticulo-

spinal projections, the raphespinal tract, is notable for inhibiting the upward transmission of signals concerned with pain. It originates in the raphe nuclei, in the midline of the medulla, and the unmyelinated serotonergic axons of the tract are lateral to the tip of the dorsal horn. The raphe nuclei are themselves stimulated by neurons in the periaqueductal gray matter of the midbrain. Electrical stimulation of the periaqueductal gray causes prompt relief of pain and has occasionally been done clinically for this purpose. A curious observation is that stimulation for a few minutes can produce analgesia lasting several hours.

2. In the **brain stem.** Large numbers of fibers descend from the somatosensory area of the cerebral cortex to the gracile and cuneate nuclei. They are presumed to influence the medial lemniscus system. Corticobulbar* fibers also end in the trigeminal sensory nuclei.

3. In the **thalamus.** The VPL and VPM nuclei project to the first somatosensory area of the cerebral cortex. These thalamic nuclei also receive input from the same cortical areas.

Clinical Abnormalities of the Somatic Sensory Pathways

The following conditions are all rather uncommon, but they serve to illustrate the relevance of neuroanatomy to clinical neurology. Figure 15-4 shows the positions of the lesions.

---

* The suffix "-bulbar" refers to the termination of axons in the brain stem. The term "corticonuclear" is sometimes used for axons of cortical neurons ending in nuclei of cranial nerves. However, many descending fibers that influence cranial nerves end near, but not within, the nuclei. The less precise term "corticobulbar" is therefore preferred.

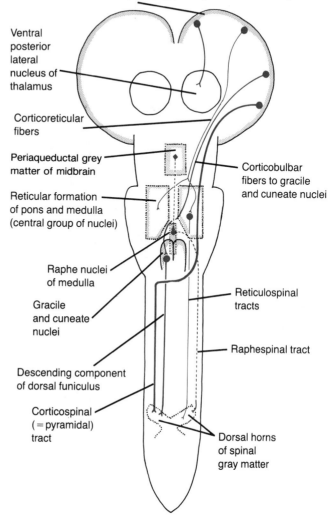

Cerebral cortex (including primary somesthetic area)

Ventral posterior lateral nucleus of thalamus

Corticoreticular fibers

Periaqueductal grey matter of midbrain

Reticular formation of pons and medulla (central group of nuclei)

Raphe nuclei of medulla

Gracile and cuneate nuclei

Descending component of dorsal funiculus

Corticospinal (= pyramidal) tract

Corticobulbar fibers to gracile and cuneate nuclei

Reticulospinal tracts

Raphespinal tract

Dorsal horns of spinal gray matter

Figure 15-3 Descending pathways that modulate the activities of the spinothalamic and medial lemniscus systems.

Hemisection of the Spinal Cord

Also known as the Brown-Séquard syndrome.*
Ipsilateral loss of proprioceptive and discrim-

inative touch sensations, contralateral loss of pain and temperature sensations. There is also a spastic paralysis of the ipsilateral musculature. The symptoms are present below the segmental level of the lesion.

* *Clinical eponyms:* Charles Édouard Brown-Séquard (1817–1894), a clinical neurologist, was a British citizen born in Mauritius of American and French parents. When old, he injected himself with extracts of simian testis and claimed that this caused rejuvenation—an early experiment in en-

docrine replacement therapy! MH Romberg (1795–1873) and Adolf Wallenberg (1862–1949) were German physicians. The word "syndrome" is defined at the end of Chapter 21.

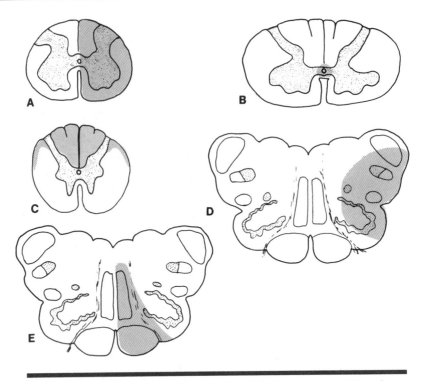

Figure 15-4   Destructive lesions (hatched areas) that cause abnormalities of somatic sensation. For discussion, see text. **(A)** Hemisection of spinal cord. **(B)** Syringomyelia. **(C)** Subacute combined degeneration of the cord. **(D)** Lateral medullary syndrome. **(E)** Medial medullary syndrome. (To identify the nuclei and tracts involved in the lesions, see figures in Chap. 7 and 8).

Syringomyelia

A cyst associated with the central canal of the spinal cord, typically in the cervical enlargement, first injures the crossing spinothalamic fibers. This causes loss of pain and temperature sensation bilaterally, at and for approximately one segment below the segmental level of the cyst. Further enlargement of the cyst can produce other symptoms.

Subacute Combined Degeneration of the Cord

Defective absorption of cyanocobalamin (vitamin B_{12}), due to inability of the stomach to secrete a glycoprotein "intrinsic factor,"

causes demyelination in the dorsal funiculi and the dorsal parts of the lateral funiculi. Discriminative tactile and proprioceptive sensations are impaired. The loss of awareness of the positions of the feet results in an ataxic (uncoordinated) gait and inability to stand upright in darkness or with the eyes shut (Romberg's sign*).

Lateral Medullary Syndrome (of Wallenberg*)

Infarction in the area shown is typically due to thrombosis of the posterior inferior cere-

* Romberg, Wallenberg: See footnote on page 113

bellar artery or one of its medullary branches. Destruction of the spinal lemniscus results in loss of pain and temperature sensation on the opposite side of the body below the neck. Destruction of the spinal trigeminal tract and nucleus causes a similar, but ipsilateral, sensory loss in the head. (See Chap. 20 for the reason, and for the effect of destruction of the nucleus ambiguus). The functions of the medial lemniscus are spared. The lesion of Wallenberg's syndrome commonly has other effects, depending on its extent. Descending fibers controlling the sympathetic nervous system pass through the area; their transection results in Horner's syndrome (see Chap. 27) ipsilaterally. Larger lesions cause cerebellar dysfunction, principally ataxia, due to involvement of the inferior cerebellar pedun-

cle. The descending motor tracts are spared by the lesion, so there is no paralysis.

Medial Medullary Syndrome

Occlusion of a small, medially directed branch of one vertebral artery can cause infarction of the region shown. Destruction of the medial lemniscus causes contralateral loss of proprioceptive and discriminative tactile sensation. There is also paralysis of half the tongue, on the side of the lesion, owing to interruption of fibers of the hypoglossal nerve. A contralateral hemiparesis (disabling weakness of the musculature of one side of the body) is attributable to destruction of motor pathways, including reticulospinal and corticospinal fibers.

Chapter 16

The Auditory System

The neural connections for hearing include the following components: (a) A sense organ of unusual complexity; (b) the cochlear division of the eighth cranial nerve; (c) an ascending central pathway containing more synaptic interruptions than the other sensory pathways and projecting bilaterally to the thalamus and cerebral cortex; (d) an extensive series of descending connections.

The Ear

The ear has three parts: the external, the middle, and the inner ear. Only part of the inner ear, the cochlea, belongs to the auditory system. The remainder of the inner ear contains the vestibular receptors for position and movement of the head.

External Ear and Middle Ear

The auricle, or pinna, serves to channel airborne sound into the earhole, or external auditory meatus. At the medial end of the external meatus is the **tympanic membrane,** or eardrum.

Medial to the eardrum is the **tympanic cavity.** This contains air, being in continuity with the nasopharynx (back of the nose) through the pharyngotympanic or eustachian* tube. The walls, roof, and floor of the tympanic cavity are made of bone, except for the tympanic

* Bartolomeo Eustachi (1513–1474) was an Italian physician and anatomist.

membrane that forms much of the lateral wall and two holes closed by collagenous membranes in the medial wall. These two holes are the **oval window** (*fenestra ovale*) and the **round window** (*fenestra rotunda*); they separate the air in the tympanic cavity from the sound-conducting liquid in the inner ear.

The tympanic membrane is connected to the oval window by a chain of three little bones known as **ossicles,** the malleus (hammer), the incus (anvil), and the stapes (stirrup). The shaping and articulation of these bones concentrate and increase the force of the vibrations of the tympanic membrane onto the smaller area of the oval window. There are also two small muscles in the middle ear. The **tensor tympani** (supplied by a branch of the trigeminal nerve) is attached to the malleus. The **stapedius** (supplied by a branch of the facial nerve) is attached to the stapes. The other ends of these muscles are anchored to the bony walls of the tympanic cavity. Contraction of the muscles limits the amplitude of movement of the little bones, providing protection against very loud sounds.

Inner Ear

The name **cochlea** alludes to the resemblance of the organ to a snail's shell excavated within the petrous part of the temporal bone of the skull. The two and one half turns of the coiled shell are lined by epithelium derived from the otic vesicle of the embryonic ectoderm. A transverse section through part of the tube (Fig. 16-1) reveals three compartments. The

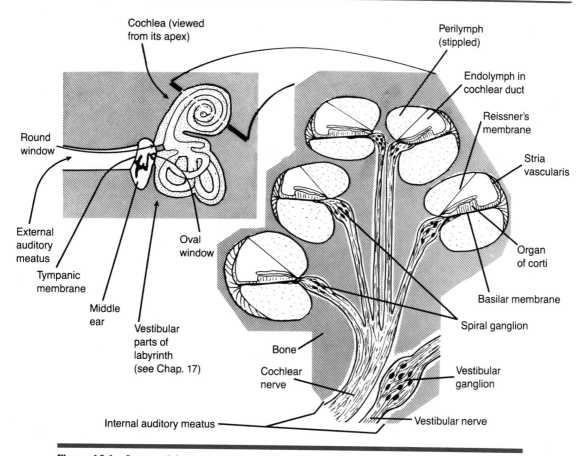

Figure 16-1 Structural features of the ear (*Left*), with details of the cochlea (*Right*).

upper and the lower contain **perilymph,** which is the sound-conducting liquid in contact with the round and oval windows. The middle compartment contains **endolymph,** a specially secreted fluid that provides a suitable environment for the receptor cells of the cochlea and also for the receptor cells of the vestibular part of the inner ear. The endolymph is secreted by the **stria vascularis** of the cochlea and is absorbed back into the blood from the **endolymphatic sac** (see Chap. 17, Fig. 17-1).

Vibrations of the stapes move the oval window and are so transmitted into the perilymph. The compression waves in the perilymph pass through the vestibular membrane

into the endolymph and cause vibrations in the basilar membrane. The pressure waves continue into the lower compartment of the perilymph to the round window. The vibration-detecting cells are in the **organ of Corti,** which rests on the basilar membrane. MA Corti (1822–1888) was the Italian histologist who described this sensory epithelium. The receptor cells, known as **hair cells,** are in four rows along the length of the organ. Each hair cell has about 100 long microvilli, known as **stereocilia,** projecting into a gelatinous membrane within the endolymph. Bending of the stereocilia occurs as a result of resonant vibration of the basilar membrane. Such vibration occurs at a characteristic position along the length of the cochlear spiral for each frequency of sound. The highest pitches are perceived near the oval window, the lowest near the apex of the cochlea.

Each hair cell is contacted at its base by both afferent and efferent nerve fibers. The afferent fiber is excited by synaptic transmission from the hair cell. The efferent endings, which are presynaptic to both the hair cells and the afferent fibers, are cholinergic. They facilitate the generation of impulses in the sensory fibers when attention is being paid to quiet sounds. The organ of Corti also contains various non-neuronal cell-types. These provide physical support and they control the chemical composition of the extracellular fluids at the apical (transducing) and basal (synaptic) poles of the hair cells.

Spiral Ganglion and Cochlear Nerve

The primary afferent neurons of the auditory system are bipolar. They are in the **spiral ganglion,** which is entombed in the bone of the central core of the cochlea, alongside the organ of Corti. The distal neurites of these bipolar cells are the fibers that receive synaptic input from the hair cells. The proximal neurites (which can unequivocally be called axons) form the **cochlear nerve.** This passes into the internal auditory meatus, the channel in the petrous bone leading into the cranial cavity. In the internal meatus, the cochlear nerve is accompanied by the vestibular nerve, the two roots of the facial nerve, and the labyrinthine artery, which supplies the inner ear.

Intracranially, the cochlear nerve occupies the angle between the pons and the cerebellum, before entering the lateral side of the medulla. The sensory fibers of the nerve end in the **dorsal and ventral cochlear nuclei,** which lie on the surface of the inferior cerebellar

peduncle. The efferent fibers of the cochlear nerve are the axons of cells in the ipsilateral and contralateral **superior olivary nuclei** (see Chap. 8; note that the superior olivary nucleus is functionally quite different from the inferior olivary complex of nuclei). The olivo-cochlear fibers leave the brain stem in the vestibular nerve. Within the internal auditory meatus, these efferent axons pass in a communicating branch to the cochlear nerve.

Ascending Central Auditory Pathways
Tonotopic Projections

The perception of each frequency of sound at its own site in the organ of Corti results in spatial separation of axons in the cochlear nerve according to pitch. This spatial separation persists throughout the nuclei and tracts of the ascending auditory pathway, to the auditory cortex. It is called **tonotopic representation;** the name is analogous to the somatotopic representation of areas of the skin in their sensory pathways.

Nuclei and Tracts

Each cochlear nerve axon bifurcates within the ventral cochlear nucleus. One branch synapses with the cells of the nucleus; the other passes dorsally to the dorsal cochlear nucleus. The **ventral cochlear nucleus** sends its axons to the **superior olivary nuclei** of *both sides.* The decussating axons constitute the **trapezoid body.** Axons from the superior olivary nucleus project rostrally in the **lateral lemniscus,** to end in the **inferior colliculus.** Some olivo-collicular fibers are ipsilateral; others cross the midline in the trapezoid body before ascending. Scattered groups of neurons within the lateral lemniscus constitute the **nucleus of the lateral lemniscus,** and provide an additional synaptic interruption. Thus the pathway from the ventral cochlear nucleus to the inferior colliculi is *bilateral* and *of variable length* (Fig. 16-2).

The axons of the cells in the **dorsal cochlear nucleus** cross the midline in the trapezoid body and then ascend in the contralateral lateral lemniscus to the inferior colliculus. This pathway is entirely crossed and consists of a single population of axons, in contrast to the pathway from the ventral cochlear nucleus described in the previous paragraph. Whereas the ventral cochlear nucleus is the source of a straightforward tonotopically organized ascending pathway, the dorsal cochlear nucleus is the site of more complicated editing of the input from the cochlea. The functional significance of the different connections of the

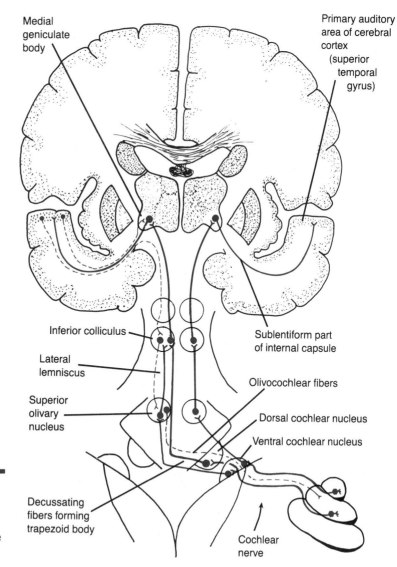

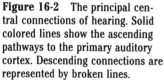

Figure 16-2 The principal central connections of hearing. Solid colored lines show the ascending pathways to the primary auditory cortex. Descending connections are represented by broken lines.

two cochlear nuclei is not yet fully understood.

The inferior colliculus projects rostrally to the **medial geniculate nucleus** of the thalamus, and this nucleus in its turn projects to the **primary auditory area** of the cerebral cortex. The primary auditory cortex is on the superior (dorsal) surface of the temporal lobe. Its tonotopic organization is such that impulses concerned with the highest frequencies of sound are received in the most medial part of the area, bordering on the insula, and impulses concerned with lower frequencies go to the lateral part of the area. The proper understanding of sounds requires the integrity of the **auditory association area,** which is posterior to the primary area. In the cerebral hemisphere that is dominant for speech and linguistic functions (the left, in most people), the auditory association cortex merges into the receptive speech area (see Chap. 22). The primary, association, and speech areas are connected by subcortical association fibers within each cerebral hemisphere, and by fibers of the corpus callosum between the two hemispheres.

Deafness

Because of the large numbers of crossed and uncrossed ascending fibers in the auditory pathway (Fig. 16-2), and also because of commissural fibers connecting the nuclei of the lateral lemnisci, the inferior colliculi, and the auditory cortical areas, *unilateral lesions above the level of the cochlear nerve and nuclei do not cause deafness.* Destructive lesions of the auditory cortex can, however, cause difficulty in localizing the origin of a sound. Studies in animals indicate that localization of sounds involves descending connections and the proper functioning of the superior olivary nucleus.

The most common causes of impaired hearing are **conduction deafness,** which is usually due to disease of the middle ear, and **perceptive deafness,** usually due to degeneration in the organ of Corti. The end of the organ of Corti nearest to the oval window is the part first damaged by prolonged exposure to loud noise. The consequence of such damage is therefore loss of the ability to hear high-pitched sounds. Similar changes often occur with aging, even without the insult of noise. A less common cause of perceptive deafness is an **acoustic neuroma.** This is a benign tumor arising from the vestibular division of cranial nerve VIII. The tumor originates in the internal auditory meatus and causes symptoms (abnormal sounds at first, and then deafness) by pressing on the cochlear nerve. As the tumor grows, it extends into the cranial cavity, in the angle between the pons and the cerebellum. There it presses on the nearby cranial nerves (VII, IX, X) and on the cerebellum, causing appropriate symptoms. If an acoustic neuroma is not diagnosed and removed, it eventually causes death by compressing the medulla.

Descending Auditory Connections

Large numbers of axons pass from the primary auditory cortex to the medial geniculate nucleus and to the inferior colliculus. The inferior colliculus sends fibers down the lateral lemniscus to the superior olivary nucleus. This nucleus is thus influenced not only by the sensory information but also by the higher centers that analyze the information. The projection from the superior olivary nucleus to the contralateral organ of Corti was described earlier in this chapter. The descending auditory connections (see Fig. 16-2) can inhibit the upward transmission of unwanted information (background noise) and enhance the attention paid to significant sounds.

Chapter 17

The Vestibular System

Sensory signals due to position and movements of the head arise in the vestibular part of the labyrinth and are sent into the brain through the vestibular division of the eighth cranial nerve. Vestibular sensation is important in making compensatory movements to maintain an erect posture, in ensuring that the direction of gaze is correct for the position of the constantly moving head, and in providing conscious awareness of position, acceleration, deceleration, and rotation. All these functions are normally supplemented by the visual system and by proprioceptive sensation from muscles and joints, especially of the lower limbs.

Labyrinth and Vestibular Receptors

The name "labyrinth" comes from the Greek, meaning a maze of underground tunnels. The **bony labyrinth** is a system of tubes and cavities hollowed out of the petrous part of the temporal bone. The **membranous labyrinth** within the bony tunnels contains the receptor organs of the vestibular and auditory systems. Chapter 16 contains a description of the receptors of the cochlea. The following description is of the vestibular apparatus (Fig. 17-1).

Saccule, Utricle, and Semicircular Ducts

Two swellings, the **saccule** and the **utricle,** are contained in the part of the bony labyrinth known as the vestibule. Three **semicircular ducts,** in planes at right angles to one another, are connected with the utricle; each duct has a bulge, the **ampulla,** at one end. The saccule, the utricle, and the semicircular ducts contain **endolymph,** a special fluid secreted by the stria vascularis of the cochlear duct, which is continuous with the cavity of the saccule. The endolymphatic duct also connects with the saccule; its other end is in the **endolymphatic sac,** from which endolymph is absorbed into the blood. The space between the endolymph-containing structures and the wall of the bony labyrinth is filled with **perilymph,** a fluid similar to the cerebrospinal fluid of the brain. The space containing perilymph is very small around the semicircular ducts. It is larger in the vestibule, and in the cochlea it forms the medium for transmission of sound on both sides of the cochlear duct.

Static Labyrinth

The sensory areas in the utricle and saccule are called **maculae** (Latin for "spots"). There is a macula in the floor of the utricle, lying horizontally, and a macula in the medial wall of the saccule, in a vertical plane parallel to the midline. Each macula contains **hair cells.** The vestibular hair cells differ from the cochlear ones in that each has a single long cilium, called a kinocilium, in addition to long microvilli or stereocilia. The ends of the kinocilia and stereocilia are embedded in a mass of ge-

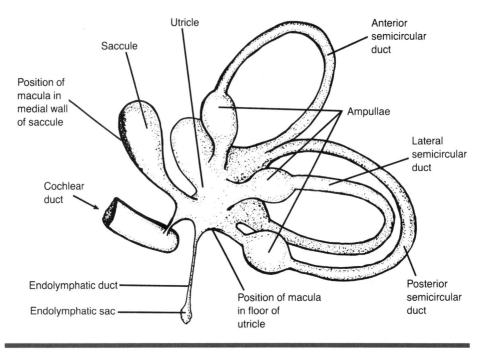

Figure 17-1   The vestibular labyrinth. (Compare with Fig. 16-1 for orientation.)

latinous material, the **otolithic membrane,** in which are suspended numerous granules. The granules, made of protein and calcium carbonate, are called **otoliths.** The name means "ear-stones." (Synonyms in common use are: otoconia, statoliths, and statoconia.) An otolithic membrane can be thought of as a small weight fixed to the floor of the utricle or side of the saccule by numerous flexible threads (Fig. 17-2). The otolithic membrane is pulled downwards by gravity. The resulting deflection of the stereocilia is transduced by the hair cells into presynaptic activity that affects the afferent nerve fibers at the bases of the cells. The nature of the response depends on the position of the head. Thus the otolithic membrane of the saccule is pulled downwards when the head is upright, and the otolithic membrane of the utricle is pulled downwards when the head is inclined forwards, back-

wards, or sideways. The maculae thus identify the direction of gravitational force. These receptors also respond to acceleration or deceleration, which will cause the otolithic membranes to swing respectively against or with the direction of movement. Movement at a constant velocity, however, does not affect these receptors.

Kinetic Labyrinth

The other receptors of the vestibular apparatus are in the ampullae of the three semicircular canals. Each resembles a macula but is on a raised crest and is surmounted not by an otolithic membrane but by a dome-shaped cupula made of gelatinous material no denser than the endolymph (Fig. 17-2). This type of receptor is a **crista ampullaris.** The stereocilia

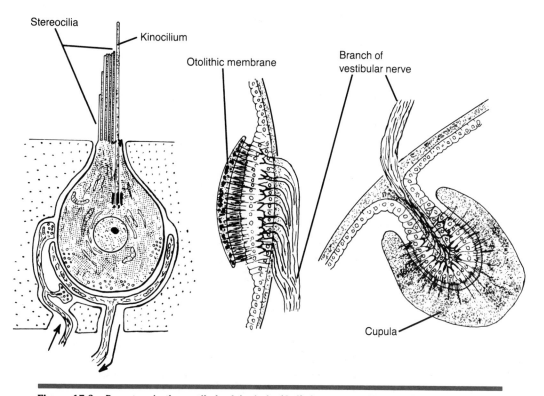

Figure 17-2   Receptors in the vestibular labyrinth. (*Left*) A receptor cell, with afferent and efferent axons. (*Center*) A macula (of the saccule or utricle). The sensory hairs are deflected by the pull of gravity on the otolithic membrane or by inertial movements during acceleration or deceleration of the head. (*Right*) Crista of the ampulla of a semicircular duct. The sensory hairs are deflected when the cupula is moved by currents in the endolymph.

of its hair cells are bent when the cupula is moved by a current in the endolymph of the semicircular duct. This occurs when the head is rotating. The fact that the three semicircular ducts are in three planes, each one perpendicular to the other two (Fig. 17-3), ensures that rotation in any direction will stimulate the crista ampullaris of at least one duct. If a person spins round quickly and stops suddenly, the endolymph will continue flowing in the direction of the rotation for a few seconds. The resultant deflection of the cupulae causes a false sensation of rotation in the opposite direction.

Innervation of Receptors

The hair cells of the vestibular apparatus are contacted by the distal neurites of the bipolar neurons of the **vestibular ganglion,** which is deep in the internal auditory meatus, near the vestibule of the labyrinth. The proximal neurites (axons) of these cells form the **vestibular nerve,** which enters the brain stem medial to the cochlear nerve and lateral to the facial nerve. Like the cochlear nerve, the vestibular nerve also contains efferent fibers. They arise from neurons in the reticular formation of the pons and terminate on the vestibular hair cells

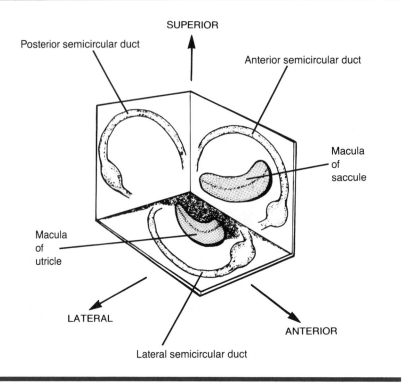

SUPERIOR

Posterior semicircular duct

Anterior semicircular duct

Macula
of
saccule

Macula
of
utricle

LATERAL

ANTERIOR

Lateral semicircular duct

Figure 17-3 A diagram to illustrate the approximate orientations of the receptors of the right vestibular apparatus. The three semicircular ducts lie in mutually perpendicular planes. One macula is horizontal, the other vertical.

and on the afferent nerve endings. The functions of these efferent fibers are unknown.

Central Vestibular Connections

Vestibular Nuclei

Most of the axons of the vestibular nerve, having entered the brain stem, end in the **vestibular nuclei.** There are four of these nuclei (superior, inferior, medial, and lateral), but for the sake of simplicity they can conveniently be lumped together as a group. A few primary afferent axons from the vestibular nerve bypass the vestibular nuclei and enter the inferior cerebellar peduncle. These direct

vestibulocerebellar fibers end in the vestibulocerebellum (see Chap. 9).

Projections From the Vestibular Nuclei
(Fig. 17-4)

The neurons of the vestibular nuclei have axons that go in four directions:

1. **To the vestibulocerebellum,** through the inferior cerebellar peduncle. As in the case of all fibers afferent to the cerebellum, these axons give off branches to a cerebellar nucleus, in this case the **fastigial nucleus,** before continuing to their sites of termination in the cerebellar cortex. The

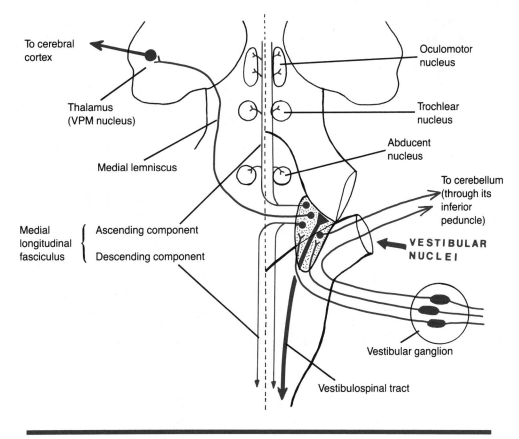

To cerebral cortex

Thalamus (VPM nucleus)

Medial lemniscus

Medial longitudinal fasciculus { Ascending component / Descending component }

Oculomotor nucleus

Trochlear nucleus

Abducent nucleus

To cerebellum (through its inferior peduncle)

VESTIBULAR NUCLEI

Vestibular ganglion

Vestibulospinal tract

Figure 17-4 Central connections of the vestibular system.

cortex of the vestibulocerebellum projects to the fastigial nucleus. The principal projection of the fastigial nucleus is to the vestibular nuclei. Thus the main action of the vestibulocerebellum is to modify the traffic of impulses in the ascending and descending fibers that leave the vestibular nuclei.

2. **The vestibulospinal tract** consists of the axons of the large neurons of one of the vestibular nuclei (the lateral vestibular nucleus; often named after the German anatomist Otto Deiters, 1834–1863). The tract descends in the ventral spinal white

matter, and its fibers end in the medial parts of the ventral horn of the spinal gray. Impulses in the vestibulospinal axons cause excitation of those motor neurons that supply the muscles that oppose gravity—the extensors of the limbs and many of the axial muscles that act on the spine. The motor neurons supplying antagonistic muscles, the flexors, are inhibited by activity in the vestibulospinal tract. Note that the vestibulospinal tract is influenced by the labyrinth and by the cerebellum, but not directly by higher levels of the neuraxis.

3. **The medial longitudinal fasciculus** contains ascending and descending fibers from the vestibular nuclei. The ascending fibers go to the motor nuclei of the oculomotor, trochlear, and abducent nerves, which supply the muscles that move the eyes. The descending fibers of the medial longitudinal fasciculus go to the cervical segments of the spinal cord; they mediate reflex movements of the neck. The medial longitudinal fasciculus also contains other populations of fibers concerned with eye movements (see Chap. 19).

4. **Pathways for conscious awareness of position** are not known with great anatomical precision. It is probable that some axons from the vestibular nuclei cross the midline and ascend in or near the medial lemniscus to the ventral posterior medial nucleus of the thalamus. This nucleus, which also relays general somatic sensation from the head, may send fibers concerned with vestibular sensation to an area of the parietal cortex adjacent to the head area of the postcentral gyrus. Clinical studies of cortical blood flow indicate, however, that vestibular sensation in man is transmitted only to a part of the temporal lobe posterior to the primary auditory area.

Vestibular Reflexes

The function of the vestibular system is to induce movements that keep the body balanced, both at rest and in motion. This is achieved partly by the actions of the vestibular nuclei on the antigravity musculature, and partly by connections through the medial longitudinal fasciculus with the muscles that move the eyes and head, thereby tending to keep the gaze fixed on a particular spot without conscious effort.

The **optokinetic reflex** is the simplest mechanism acting to conserve the direction of gaze.

When the head rotates in one direction, the two eyes move through an equal angle in the opposite direction. This reflex requires the integrity of the vestibular apparatus, nerves, and nuclei, the medial longitudinal fasciculus, and cranial nerves III, IV, and VI. In conscious people the optokinetic reflex is apparent only with small angular rotations because larger movements are associated with voluntary shifting of the point of fixation of gaze.

In a patient whose brain stem is functioning normally but whose cerebral hemispheres are not working, an exaggerated optokinetic reflex known as the "doll's eyes phenomenon" is observed.

The **caloric reflex** is a useful clinical test of vestibular function. With the patient's head reclining at 60° from vertical, the external auditory meatus is irrigated with warm (42°–44°C) water. This warms the endolymph in the lateral semicircular duct, setting up a convection current. The upward flow of warmed endolymph deflects the crista ampullaris as it would if the head were rotating towards the side being tested. Accordingly, the eyes slowly turn towards the opposite side. This movement is followed by a rapid voluntary movement of the eyes back toward the side being tested. The sequence of eye movements is then repeated.

Alternating slow and rapid movements of the eyes are called **nystagmus** (which in Greek means nodding off to sleep). Unfortunately it is conventional to identify a nystagmus by the direction of the fast correcting movement rather than by the slow reflex movement. Thus irrigation of the right ear with warm water normally causes a "right nystagmus."

Disease of the membranous labyrinth causes **vertigo,** a false sensation of rotation, accompanied by nystagmus. This may be due to abnormal stimulation of the receptors or, if the receptors have been put out of action, to the unbridled effects of the input from the contralateral labyrinth. Destruction of one labyrinth causes vertigo and nystagmus, with the rapid movement toward the opposite side. The patient falls or turns to the side of the nonfunctional labyrinth because the contralateral vestibulospinal tract is overactive. Eventually the vertigo from a destroyed labyrinth or a transected VIIIth cranial nerve subsides, and the central nervous system adapts to having the input of only one vestibular labyrinth. Transient vertigo is often due to virus infections of the labyrinth or of the vestibular ganglion. **Ménière's disease** (first recognized by Prosper Ménière, 1801–1862, a French physician) is a more serious condition. Excessive production of endolymph causes unduly high pressure (endolymphatic hydrops) in the membranous labyrinth. Stimulation of the receptors is followed by their destruction, which leads eventually to loss of both cochlear and vestibular function.

There are connections (not shown in Fig. 17-4) of the vestibular nuclei with the reticular formation of the medulla. The reticular formation has many functions, including involvement in the activities of the internal organs of the abdomen. Excessive stimulation of the vestibular receptors in susceptible people causes unpleasant sensations that would otherwise be attributed to disease of the stomach, and vomiting may occur as a result. This condition is **motion sickness.** Its pathological physiology is poorly understood, and it is not known why some people are susceptible but others are not.

Chapter 18

The Visual System

Vision involves the collection by the eyes of ordered optical pictures of the outside world and transduction of the images into corresponding patterns of nerve impulses. The neural activity is analyzed by the brain to provide interpretations of what is consciously seen and to use the visual information unconsciously for the maintenance of steady postures and movements.

The Eye

It is assumed that the reader has an elementary understanding of how a mammalian eye works. Figure 18-1 shows some anatomical and optical features pertinent to the neural mechanisms of vision. The following points are noteworthy:

1. The real image produced by light falling on the retina is inverted.
2. In man, both eyes face forward, so that images of most of the territory in front of the face are formed on both retinas.
3. Because of the inversion of images and the forward-facing eyes, the left half of the visual field is projected onto the right half of each retina, and *vice versa.*
4. The retina and optic nerve are parts of the central nervous system, being derived from the embryonic diencephalon.
5. The eye also contains peripheral nerves, which enter as ciliary nerves that pierce the sclera. Sensory fibers are branches of the ophthalmic division of the trigeminal nerve. Autonomic axons are from the superior cervical ganglion and the ciliary ganglion.
6. The ophthalmic artery is a branch of the internal carotid artery. The central artery of the retina, a branch of the ophthalmic artery, runs in the center of the optic nerve. It branches lie on the inside of the retina. The central retinal vein drains into the ophthalmic vein, which drains into the cavernous sinus.

Retina

Focused images are detected and partly analyzed in the retina. The analysis causes the retina's output of impulses to be more than a faithful copy of the optical image. The patterning of impulses in the axons of the optic nerve carries additional information, generated in the retina, concerning contrast at the edges of objects, directions of alignment of edges, moving objects, and colors. These functions are possible because of neuronal circuitry within the retina. There are three types of neurons: **Photoreceptors, interneurons,** and principal cells. Neurons of the last-named type are called **ganglion cells;** their axons form the optic nerve and end in the brain. The radial glial cells of the retina (Fig. 18-2) are known as **Müller cells,** after Heinrich Müller (1820–1864), a German anatomist. There are

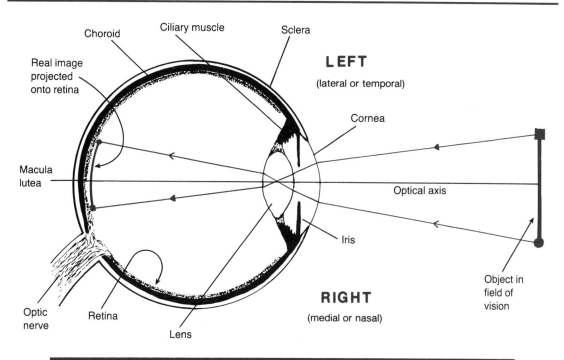

Figure 18-1   Anatomy and optics of the eye. A horizontal section through the left eye, viewed from above, showing the focusing of a real, inverted image on the retina. Behind the lens, the eyeball is filled by the **vitreous body,** which is transparent and gelatinous. The space between the lens and the cornea is occupied by **aqueous humor,** a liquid secreted by the **ciliary processes** (anterior to ciliary muscle) and absorbed into veins at the angle between the iris and the cornea. The **posterior chamber** of the eye is between the lens and the iris; the **anterior chamber** is between the iris and the cornea. The cells of the **choroid** contain a pigment, melanin, which prevents reflections of light within the eyeball.

astrocytes in the nerve fiber layer of the retina, but usually no oligodendrocytes, because the axons remain unmyelinated until they enter the optic nerve. Rarely there are some bundles of myelinated axons in the normal human retina; they are visible through the ophthalmoscope as white streaks radiating from the optic disc.

Photoreceptors

Light must pass through the transparent layers of principal cells and interneurons before it is detected (Fig. 18-2). The outermost layer of the retina, the pigment epithelium, pre-

vents scattering of light among the photoreceptors. Each photoreceptor cell has two parts. The **inner segment,** which contains the nucleus and other organelles of a neuron, is joined to the outer segment by a thin strand of cytoplasm. The **outer segment** contains membranous discs. The discs carry the pigment that absorbs light and responds with a chemical change that affects the presynaptic part of the surface membrane of the inner segment. There are two types of photoreceptor, the rod and the cone. The names allude (rather inaccurately) to the shapes of the outer segment of the cells.

Rods are most abundant in the peripheral

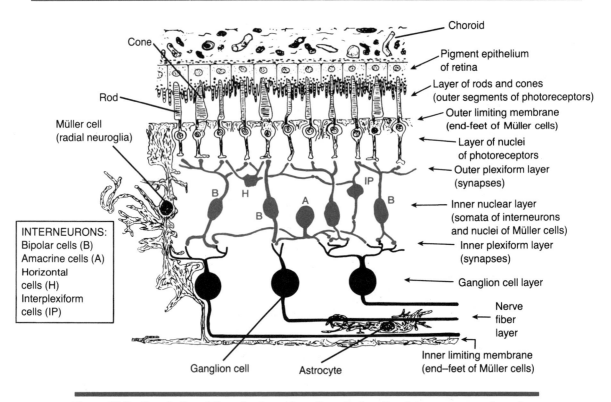

Cone

Rod

Müller cell
(radial neuroglia)

INTERNEURONS:
Bipolar cells (B)
Amacrine cells (A)
Horizontal
cells (H)
Interplexiform
cells (IP)

Choroid

Pigment epithelium
of retina

Layer of rods and cones
(outer segments of photoreceptors)

Outer limiting membrane
(end-feet of Müller cells)

Layer of nuclei
of photoreceptors

Outer plexiform layer
(synapses)

Inner nuclear layer
(somata of interneurons
and nuclei of Müller cells)

Inner plexiform layer
(synapses)

Ganglion cell layer

Nerve
fiber
layer

Inner limiting membrane
(end–feet of Müller cells)

Ganglion cell   Astrocyte

Figure 18-2   Organization of the retina in a schematic vertical section. Interneurons are shown in
color. In reality the retina is packed with cells, and there is hardly any extracellular space. The *ten
layers* of the retina are listed at the right-hand side of the figure. The potential space between the
pigment epithelium and the layer of rods and cones is the "optic ventricle," the remnant of the cavity
of the optic vesicle (see Fig. 5-5).

parts of the retina, and they are optimally effective in weak light. Rods cannot distinguish colors. The central part of the retina, in the optical axis of the cornea and lens, is called the **macula lutea** (Latin for "yellow spot," from its ophthalmoscopic appearance; the peripheral retina has an orange–red color). **Cones** are most abundant in the macula, especially in its central spot, the **fovea centralis** (central depression, where the retina is at its thinnest). Cones work best in bright light. There are three types of cones, with pigments that absorb red, green, or blue light. A mixture of these colors is perceived as white by the human eye.

The surface of a photoreceptor has a membrane potential of −30 mV in darkness. This permits continuous leakage of the neurotransmitter from the presynaptic sites at the inner end of the inner segment (see Chap. 3). When the outer segment is illuminated, the membrane potential is restored to a resting level of about −70 mV, with consequent prevention of the release of the transmitter. Thus light *inhibits* the activity of the photoreceptors.

Retinal Neurons and Intrinsic Circuitry

The inner segments of the rods and cones are presynaptic to the dendrites of the **bipolar cells.** The axons of the bipolar cells are presynaptic to the **ganglion cells.** Although the main cytoplasmic processes of the bipolar cell are called "dendrite" and "axon," these cells do not develop action potentials, so in a physiological sense both processes are dendrites. Signalling within such cells is by the propagation of graded changes in the membrane potential. The same is true of the other types of retinal interneuron. The ganglion cells are the only cells in the retina that transmit ordinary nerve impulses.

Electrophysiological investigations have revealed two major types of bipolar cell in the retina. *Depolarizing bipolars* develop increased membrane potential in response to light. In other words, the reduced amount of transmitter from the photoreceptors causes postsynaptic excitation. The *hyperpolarizing bipolars* are inhibited when they receive smaller amounts of transmitter from their afferent photoreceptors. This second type of bipolar neuron is made active, therefore, by the dark parts of an image projected onto the retina. Both types of bipolar cell are excitatory to ganglion cells.

Several types of ganglion cells are recognized. The *on* types are postsynaptic to depolarizing bipolars, so they generate action potentials in response to illumination. *Off* ganglion calls are postsynaptic to hyperpolarizing cells, so they produce impulses in response to darkness. There are ganglion cells of *on* and *off* type that respond to continuous light or dark, or to changes in the intensity of the incident light. There is considerable convergence of photoreceptors upon bipolar neurons, though each photoreceptor is presynaptic to both types of bipolar cell. There is further convergence of bipolars upon smaller numbers of ganglion cells. The greatest convergence is in the peripheral retina, and the number of photoreceptors per ganglion cell decreases toward the center. In the middle of the fovea centralis, there is 1:1:1 transmission from photoreceptors to bipolars to ganglion cells. This small area has the highest capacity for resolution, known as **visual acuity.**

The bipolar cells form part of the direct sequence of retinal neurons. There are also three other types of retinal interneuron. **Horizontal cells** are postsynaptic to photoreceptors and presynaptic to bipolar cells, which they inhibit. Activity of the horizontal cells causes reduced activity (that is, higher membrane potentials) in bipolar cells immediately outside an area of the retina that is responding strongly to either light or darkness. The result is a reduced frequency of impulses generated by ganglion cells beside the edge of an image. The brain thus receives signals that emphasize contrasts. **Amacrine cells** modulate synaptic transmission from bipolar to ganglion cells. The name "amacrine" comes from Greek roots that imply an absence of length, because the short dendrites all emerge from one side of the cell. The **interplexiform cells** are postsynaptic to amacrines and presynaptic to horizontal and bipolar cells, thereby providing a link between the two main synaptic layers of the retina.

Optic Nerves, Chiasma, and Tracts

The axons of the ganglion cells travel in the **optic nerve** to the brain. On the ventral (inferior) surface of the hypothalamus, the two optic nerves meet and there is decussation of some of their fibers in the **optic chiasma.** The axons emerging from the chiasma continue in the **optic tracts** to sites of termination in the thalamus and midbrain. In laboratory animals, some optic axons turn dorsally at the chiasma to terminate in the anterior hypothalamus. It is not known if a retino-hypothalamic connection exists in man.

The axons that cross the midline in the optic chiasma are those from the medial (or "nasal") half of the retina. Axons from the lateral ("temporal") half of the retina do not cross; they continue into the ipsilateral optic tract. The line of separation between "lateral" and "medial" passes through the fovea centralis. *The partial decussation causes each half of each retina to project into the optic tract of the same side.*

Axons of the optic tract go to three places. Most end in the **lateral geniculate body** of the thalamus.* Others end in the **superior colliculus** and in a more rostral part of the midbrain, the **pretectal area.** The pathway to and beyond the lateral geniculate body is the one for conscious sight. The pretectal area is involved in the reflex responses of the pupil. The superior colliculi are involved in the control of the muscles that move the eyes.

Pathway for Conscious Vision

Most of the axons of the optic tract end in the **lateral geniculate body** of the thalamus. (The precise site is the *dorsal nucleus of the lateral geniculate body.*) The neurons in this thalamic nucleus have axons that travel in the retrolentiform part of the internal capsule to the **cerebral cortex around the calcarine sulcus** on the medial surface of the occipital lobe. This primary visual area is called the **striate cortex,** because the afferent fibers form a white

* In animals small numbers of optic axons end in the pulvinar (see Chap. 10), which also receives afferent fibers from the superior colliculus and the pretectal area. The nuclei of the pulvinar project to the parietal, temporal, and occipital lobes of the cerebral cortex. It is reasonable to suppose that these accessory visual connections also exist in man, but their functions are not known.

stripe that can be seen with the unaided eye. The stripe is known as the line of Gennari, after Francesco Gennari (1750–1796), the Italian medical student who first noticed and described it.

There is precise **retinotopic organization** throughout the pathway from the retina to the primary visual cortex. Thus specific parts of the retina are connected with specific regions of the lateral geniculate body and occipital cortex. Even the fibers in the optic nerve, the optic tract, and the geniculocalcarine tract are retinotopically organized.

The projections of the left and right halves of the retinas to the same sides of the cerebrum were mentioned earlier in this chapter. Two other principles govern the distribution of fibers from each pair of half-retinas to the occipital cortex.

1. The upper halves of the retinas project to the upper lips of the calcarine sulci; the lower halves project to the lower lips of the calcarine sulci.
2. The fibers dealing with the macula lutea are segregated from those concerned with peripheral vision. Each half-macula projects to the most posterior part of the striate cortex, near the occipital pole of the hemisphere. Some geniculocalcarine fibers loop forward into the temporal lobe before turning back toward the occipital cortex. These fibers constitute Meyer's loop;* they carry information from the lower halves of the retinas.

The retinotopic projections are summarized in Figure 18-3. *It is important to remember that images on the retina are inverted.* Thus each half of the visual field is projected to the contralateral thalamus and cortex, and the upper and lower halves of the *visual fields*

* Adolph Meyer (1866–1950) was an American psychiatrist who recognized the diagnostic significance of visual field defects in destructive lesions involving the temporal lobe.

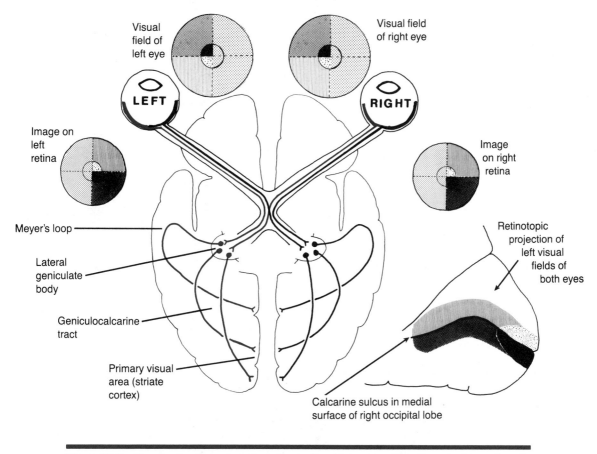

Figure 18-3   The visual pathway from the retina to the striate cortex. Note the optical inversion of the visual fields and the retinotopic projection in which fibers concerned with macular vision are segregated from those for peripheral vision.

project respectively to the lower and upper lips of the calcarine sulcus. The fibers of Meyer's loop deal with the contralateral upper quadrants of the visual fields of both eyes.

The primary visual cortex cannot, by itself, provide full recognition and understanding of the images on the retina. Connections with the surrounding **visual association area,** which accounts for most of the remaining cortex of the occipital lobe, are needed for the proper conscious appreciation of things that are seen (see Chap. 22). The occipital cortex is also important in the control of movements of the eyes that occur with the unconscious fixation

of the gaze on stationary or moving objects (see Chap. 19). The posterior part of the **parietal lobe** is necessary for recognition of the positions in space of objects that have been seen and identified, and for the performance of visually guided movements. Another visual association area is the cortex of the lateral part of the inferior (ventral) surface of the **temporal lobe,** where visual memories may be stored. The inferior temporal cortex is connected by long association fibers with the cortex of the occipital lobe.

The analysis of information in the primary visual cortex has been studied in great detail by recording from microelectrodes and by tracing with [^{14}C]2-deoxyglucose, a marker of actively working cells. Vertical columns of neurons in the cortex respond selectively to such stimuli as dark/light contrast, angle of orientation of linear objects, and lines that meet at 90° angles. In addition, the columns of neurons receiving information from the ipsilateral, the contralateral, or both eyes are arranged in a pattern of stripes across the calcarine cortex. The Nobel prize for Physiology or Medicine was awarded in 1981 to D.H. Hubel, born in Canada but now an American citizen, and to T.N. Wiesel, a Swede. Both are professors of neurobiology at Harvard. They shared the prize with R.W. Sperry (see Chap. 22). Hubel and Wiesel discovered the functional parcellations of the visual cortex, finding that anatomically distinct columns of cortical neurons responded to different and functionally meaningful appearances in the visual fields. It is likely that the whole cerebral cortex is filled with comparable columns of neurons, each attuned to a particular code of impulses that might result from a significant sensory stimulus or from a command originating elsewhere in the brain. Hubel and Wiesel have also shown that the development of cortical cell columns that recognize patterns is partly acquired through visual experience in early postnatal life. It is well known that diseases of the eyes in babies must be treated in early childhood if useful vision is to be attained.

Abnormalities of the Visual System

Visual Fields

The visual fields can be tested crudely by **confrontation,** in which the limits of the patient's peripheral vision are compared with the presumably normal visual fields of the physician. **Perimetry** is a more precise method of plotting the visual fields. The patient's head is kept still in a chinrest, with the gaze fixed on a small, bright object. The visual fields are explored with a small movable light, and the angular coordinates are plotted on specially printed graph paper. The eyes are tested separately, and the result is a pair of diagrams showing the shapes of the visual fields of the two eyes. A normal visual field consists of two roughly circular outlines. The lower and medial (nasal) part of each circle is missing, because the bridge of the nose obstructs the passage of light to the upper, outer edge of each retina.

Inability to see may be due to disease in either the eye or the brain. The most common eye disease to affect the visual field is chronic glaucoma. The raised intraocular pressure in this disease injures the retina, and the usual result is a blind patch (*scotoma*) in the middle of the visual field of the affected eye. Degeneration of the maculae, with small but disabling central scotomata, is common in the aged.

The abnormalities of the visual fields due to disease of the central nervous system can be deduced from simple facts of neuroanatomy. In order to test his or her understanding of the retinotopic projections, the student should try to answer the questions posed in Figure 18-4. A simple plan of the pathway, which need be no bigger than a postage stamp, is a useful *aide memoire* for clinical problems. Even in a tiny diagram (inset in Fig. 18-4), it is important to indicate that the optical system of the eye produces an inverted image on the retina.

Cortical Lesions

Unilateral damage to the primary visual cortex is typically associated with macular sparing, in which the central part of the contralateral visual field is not blind. The sparing is probably an artifact of testing caused by small compensatory movements of the eyes.

Destructive lesions of the association cortex

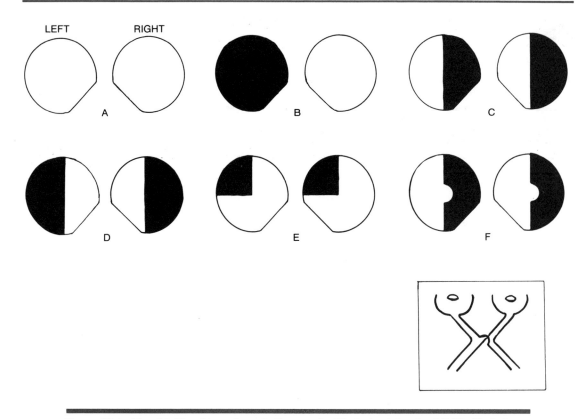

Figure 18-4   Visual field problems. In each diagram, the *blind* part of the *visual field* is black. Locate the lesions in the visual pathway.
Answers:

(F) Destruction of left visual cortex, with macular sparing.
(E) Destruction of Meyer's loop in right temporal lobe.
(D) Lesion in the midline of the optic chiasma.
(C) Transection of the left optic tract, or destruction of left lateral geniculate body.
(B) Left eye blind, for any reason.
(A) Normal

of the occipital and neighboring part of the parietal lobe have to be bilateral to cause difficulty in the mental interpretation of the visual image, because the cortices of the two sides are connected by the corpus callosum. Bilateral lesions cause difficulty in recognizing shapes and colors. Unilateral destruction of the posterior part of the parietal lobe (especially of the right hemisphere) sometimes causes the patient not to notice objects in the contralateral halves of the visual fields (see Chap. 22).

Failure to recognize familiar sites is one consequence of ablation of both temporal lobes. A similar effect can follow bilateral destruction of the inferior longitudinal fasciculus, which connects the occipital with the temporal cortex. Electrical stimulation of the inferior surface of the temporal lobe in conscious neurosurgical patients evokes awareness of remembered visual scenes. Similar hallucinations occur in the initial stages of epileptic seizures that begin in this part of the temporal lobe.

Chapter 19

Eye Movements

and Visual Reflexes

Movements of the eyes have to be accurately coordinated, for if they are not the brain will fail to fuse the patterns of nerve impulses signalling the images on the two retinas, and the advantages of binocular vision will be largely lost. When gazing at a distant scene, the two eyes move together (**conjugate movement**); when looking at a near object, the eyes look toward one another (**convergence**).

The **extraocular muscles** are striated skeletal muscles. Inside the eye are smooth muscles. The **iris** contains the dilator and the sphincter of the pupil. The **ciliary muscle,** attached to the suspensory ligament (or zonule) of the lens, is used for focusing.

Extraocular Muscles and Their Actions

The six extraocular muscles originate around the foramen through which the optic nerve enters the cranium and are inserted into the sclera. The four **rectus muscles,** superior, inferior, medial, and lateral, insert above, below, medial, and lateral to the cornea. They pull the eye so that it looks up, down, medially, and laterally, respectively (see Fig. 19-1). The two **oblique muscles,** inferior and superior, have less obvious actions. Acting in isolation they would pull on the eye to make it look up-and-out or down-and-out, respectively, because the tendons are inserted behind the equator of the eyeball. No extraocular muscles act in isolation, however. The most conspicuous consequence of synergy is that the superior oblique collaborates with the medial rectus and therefore makes the eyeball look downward and inward.

The extraocular muscles are supplied with **motor fibers** by cranial nerves III, IV, and VI, the oculomotor, trochlear, and abducent nerves. Nerves IV and VI each supply only one muscle, the superior oblique and lateral rectus, respectively. Nerve III supplies all the other extraocular muscles and the **levator palpebrae superioris,** the muscle that elevates the upper eyelid. Motor units in the eye-moving muscles are very small; each neuron supplies only about 10 muscle fibers. Thus these muscles are controlled with great precision. **Proprioceptive endings** are supplied, in laboratory animals, by sensory axons from the trigeminal nerve, though some sensory fibers may enter the brain stem through nerves III, IV, and VI. In addition to motor axons, the oculomotor nerve contains preganglionic parasympathetic fibers.

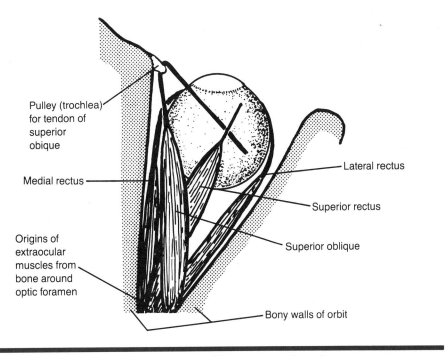

Pulley (trochlea) for tendon of superior obique

Medial rectus

Origins of extraocular muscles from bone around optic foramen

Lateral rectus

Superior rectus

Superior oblique

Bony walls of orbit

Figure 19-1   Some of the muscles acting on the right eye, as seen from above.

Oculomotor Nerve (Fig. 19-2)

Anatomy

The oculomotor nerve emerges from the midbrain (Chap. 8) and tranverses the subarachnoid space, passing over the free edge of the tontorium cerebelli (Chap. 28). After passing through the cavernous sinus (Chap. 28, Chap. 29), the nerve enters the orbit through the superior orbital fissure. Branches go to *five muscles:* Superior rectus, inferior rectus, medial rectus, inferior oblique, and levator palpebrae superioris. The last-named muscle also contains some smooth muscle fibers, supplied with sympathetic fibers from the superior cervical ganglion (see Chap. 27). The preganglionic parasympathetic fibers of the oculomotor nerve travel in the branch to the in-ferior oblique, and then in a communicating nerve to the ciliary ganglion.

Functional Components

The **somatic motor** axons arise from cells in the **oculomotor nucleus,** which is in the rostral part of the midbrain.

There is a subnucleus for each muscle supplied by the oculomotor nerve. The axons from the subnucleus supplying the superior rectus cross the midline and leave the brainstem in the contralateral nerve. The levator palpebrae superioris is supplied bilaterally by a subnucleus that straddles the midline. The other three muscles are innervated by ipsilateral subnuclei. The motor axons pass ventrally through the tegmentum (including the

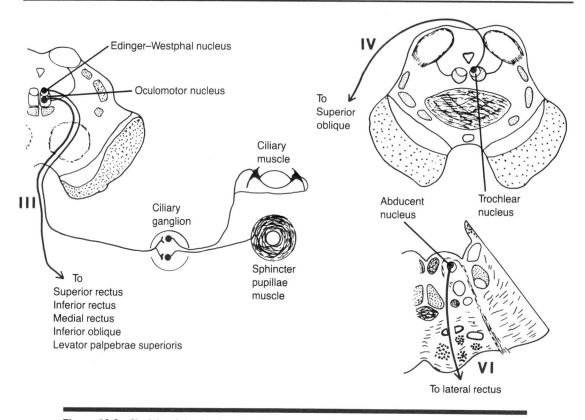

Figure 19-2   Nuclei and destinations of the oculomotor, trochlear, and abducent nerves. The post-ganglionic parasympathetic neurons controlled by the oculomotor nerve are also shown.

red nucleus) to reach the medial surface of the cerebral peduncle.

The **preganglionic autonomic** (parasympathetic) axons arise from the **Edinger–Westphal nucleus,** a rather indistinct group of cells dorsal to the main oculomotor complex of nuclei. The nucleus is named after two German clinical neurologists, Ludwig Edinger, 1885–1918, and Karl Westphal, 1833–1890. Axons from their nucleus pass ventrally into the ipsilateral oculomotor nerve and terminate in the **ciliary ganglion,** which is in the posterior part of the orbit, close to the optic nerve. The neurons in the ciliary ganglion have axons that pass anteriorly in the **short ciliary nerves.** These nerves go through the connective tissue around the optic nerve and then over the surface of the sclera. They pierce the sclera just behind the margin of the cornea and are distributed within the eye to the **ciliary muscle** and the **sphincter pupillae.**

When the ciliary muscle contracts, it pulls the origin of the suspensory ligament forward, making a smaller ring and thus lowering the tension in the radially oriented fibers. Tension in the suspensory ligament makes the lens thinner and flatter (long focal length). Relaxation of the tension, brought about by contraction of the ciliary muscle, allows the lens to assume a fatter, more nearly spherical, form (short focal length). Assumption of spherical form is an intrinsic property of the lens, which can be though of as a transparent jelly contained in an elastic membrane. With increasing age the lens gets tougher, and accommodation becomes a slower process.

The sphincter pupillae, formed by the circular muscle fibers of the iris, is also called the "constrictor pupillae." Constriction of the pupil has two purposes. It protects the retina from damage that would occur in bright light, and it improves the optical properties of the lens by allowing only the central part to be used.

Trochlear and Abducent Nerves

The fourth and sixth cranial nerves are the easiest ones to understand. Each has a single component, somatic motor, and each supplies one muscle.

Trochlear Nerve (Fig. 19-2)

The axons constituting this nerve arise from neurons in the **trochlear nucleus,** which is in the caudal part of the midbrain. The axons course dorsally and caudally, then cross the midline, in the superior medullary velum. Having decussated, the axons leave the dorsal surface of the brain stem. The trochlear nerve passes beside the midbrain, traverses the cavernous sinus, enters the orbit through the superior orbital fissure, and supplies the **superior oblique muscle.**

The trochlear nerve is unique in emerging from the dorsal surface of the brain stem. It does this in all vertebrate animals (see Chap. 12, Fig. 12-5).

Abducent Nerve (Fig. 19-2)

The axons of this nerve are those of neurons in the **abducent nucleus,** which is in the caudal part of the pons. The nucleus is close to fibers that will become the facial nerve and to the paramedian pontine reticular formation, a region involved in conjugate eye movements (explained later in this chapter). The motor axons pass ventrally and leave the brain stem immediately rostral to the pyramid.

The abducent nerve courses rostrally through the subarachnoid space and the cavernous sinus, and passes into the orbit through the superior orbital fissure, and supplies the **lateral rectus muscle.** The sole function of this muscle is to abduct the eye, making it look to the side, hence the name of the nerve.

Saccadic and Smooth Pursuit Movements of the Eyes

The eyes make two kinds of conjugate movements. **Saccadic movements** (or saccades) are those that shift the direction of gaze from one object to another; typically this is a voluntary act. These fast movements, which are made accurately without overshooting, are the only ones that can be done without following an object moving through the field of vision. The other type of conjugate movement is known as **smooth pursuit** or tracking, and it serves to keep the fovea of the retina aimed at a moving object in the visual field. If the target of visual fixation moves out of view, a saccadic movement brings the gaze to bear on another object. *Slow conjugate movements cannot be made voluntarily if nothing in the visual field is moving.* Movement of the head is associated with smooth pursuit movements that tend to hold the image of the target of fixation on the fovea. Of course, it is a voluntary act to follow a moving object with the eyes, but the volition relates more to the sensory function of looking than to the motor function of slowly moving the eyes.

Nystagmus (see Chap. 17) involves slow movements, resembling tracking movements, in the slow phase induced by the optokinetic reflex. The rapid movements of nystagmus are saccades. **Convergence** of the eyes, though not a conjugate movement, is comparable to smooth pursuit, because the eyes are aimed at a target brought into the visual field at short range.

All movements of the eyes are due to stimulation of the motor neurons that supply the contracting muscles, accompanied by inhibition of the neurons that innervate antagonistic muscles. Thus looking to the left requires contraction of the left lateral rectus and of the right medial rectus, while the motor neurons for the right lateral rectus and left medial rectus are inhibited. One mechanism of inhibition resides in the **inhibitory internuclear neurons.** These are neurons in the nuclei of cranial nerves III, IV, and VI that send their axons to nuclei and subnuclei that supply the antagonistic muscles. The axons of the inhibitory internuclear neurons course through the medial longitudinal fasciculus.

Gaze Centers in the Brain Stem

Certain regions in the brain stem are called gaze centers because they are necessary for conjugate movements of the eyes. The gaze centers are influenced by the retina, the superior colliculus, and the cerebral cortex.

The **paramedian pontine reticular formation** is the *center for lateral gaze*. It is also known as the PPRF and as the parabducent nucleus. Activity of neurons in the PPRF causes the eyes to look to the same side. A destructive lesion there results in inability to look to the same side.

In the **rostral part of the midbrain,** there are *centers for upward and downward gaze*. Tiny destructive lesions close to the periaqueductal gray can cause paralysis of either upward or downward conjugate eye movements.

In addition to the gaze centers, several other populations of neurons are involved in moving the eyes. These include the superior colliculus, the pretectal area, several nuclei in the rostral midbrain (interstitial nucleus of Cajal,[*] nucleus of Darkschewitsch,[†] nucleus of the posterior commissure, rostral interstitial nucleus of the medial longitudinal fasciculus; these are collectively known as the accessory oculomotor nuclei), the vestibular and perihypoglossal nuclei in the medulla, and the vestibulocerebellum.

Descending Pathway for Voluntary Saccadic Eye Movements

An area of cerebral cortex on the lateral surface of the frontal lobe is known as the **frontal eye field,** because electrical stimulation there causes conjugate movement of the eyes to the contralateral side. Destruction of the frontal eye field causes conjugate deviation of the eyes toward the side of the lesion. The pathway from the frontal cortex to the oculomotor, trochlear, and abducent nuclei is not certainly known in man. The descending pathway crosses the midline in the midbrain and includes the paramedian pontine reticular formation and the medial longitudinal fasciculus (Fig. 19-3).

Pathways Controlling Smooth Pursuit Movements

The frontal eye field is not involved in tracking movements. Thus a patient who cannot make voluntary saccadic movements in re-

---

[*] See Chapter 13 for a biographical footnote on Ramon y Cajal. His surname is often incorrectly shortened to Cajal, especially in eponyms.
[†] LO Darkschewitsch (1859–1925) was a Russian clinical neurologist.

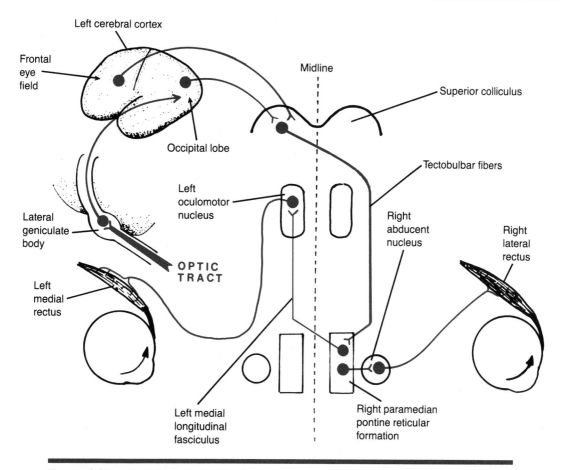

Figure 19-3   Some of the neuronal circuitry that controls conjugate movement of the eyes to the right. For a *voluntary saccadic movement*, the pathway begins in the frontal eye field. For a *smooth pursuit movement*, the pathway begins in the retina and in the occipital cortex.

sponse to a request to "look to the left" or "look up," may have no difficulty in following a moving object such as the physician's hand or face. The cortex used for smooth pursuit movements is that of most of the occipital lobe. This **occipital eye field** is coextensive with the primary visual area together with much of the visual association cortex.

The descending pathway for smooth pursuit movements is probably similar to that for saccadic movements, but the eyes and the vestibular system are also involved (Fig. 19-3).

Accommodation and Convergence

Three events occur when the gaze is shifted from a distant to a near target: *Convergence* of the eyes, *focusing* of the lens, and *constriction* of the pupil.

The pathways involved in convergence are

poorly understood. They are probably similar to those for smooth pursuit movement, because convergence requires the integrity of the occipital, but not of the frontal, eye fields. The paramedian pontine reticular formation, however, is not needed for convergence. The existence of a convergence center in the midbrain has been postulated.

The central pathways mediating focusing and pupillary constriction in the accomodating eye are likewise largely unknown. The superior colliculus and its retinal afferent fibers are almost certainly involved. The pathway for accommodation does *not* include the pretectal area, and thus differs from that of the light reflex.

Light Reflex

This clinically important reflex consists of constriction of the pupil when a light is shone into the eye. At the same time, the pupil of the other eye also constricts, even though it has not been illuminated. The latter constriction is called the **consensual response.** The pathways are illustrated in Figure 19-4, which will enable the student to determine the sites of lesions that affect the light reflex. Preganglionic parasympathetic fibers are near the surface of the trunk of the oculomotor nerve, so if the nerve is compressed these fibers are adversely affected sooner than the somatic motor fibers.

Vestibulo-ocular Reflexes

The connections between the vestibular nuclei and the nuclei of cranial nerves III, IV, and VI have been described in Chapter 17. The most important abnormal vestibulo-ocular reflex is **nystagmus,** described in Chapter 17 and also mentioned earlier in this chapter.

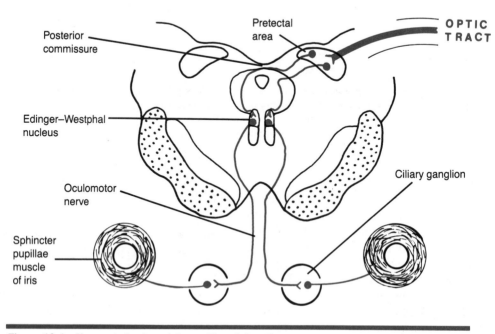

Figure 19-4   Neuronal circuitry of the pupillary light reflex.

Disorders of the Oculomotor System

Derangements of movement of the eyes may be due to malfunction of the cerebral cortex, the brain stem, or the cranial nerves that supply the extraocular muscles.

Cortical Lesions Affecting Conjugate Gaze

Destruction of the frontal eye field causes deviation of both eyes toward the side of the lesion. Voluntary (saccadic) movements of the eyes away from the side of the cortical lesion cannot be made. Commonly this condition is due to ischemic damage to a larger area of cerebral cortex, which also includes the motor and premotor areas, with consequent paralysis of the limbs and lower half of the face on the contralateral side. The deviated eyes look away from the paralyzed side of the body.

A large destructive lesion in one occipital lobe causes inability to make smooth pursuit movements away from the side of the lesion, although voluntary saccades are unaffected. If the lesion includes the striate cortex, there is also blindness in the contralateral halves of the visual fields of both eyes.

Lesions in the Brain Stem That Affect Gaze

A lesion that destroys the abducent nucleus is almost certain to involve the PPRF of the same side too. The result is paralysis of the ipsilateral lateral rectus, with permanent medial deviation of the affected eye, together with inability to move the contralateral eye further medially than when it is looking straight forward. This condition may be contrasted with a lesion involving the motor axons of the abducent nerve, either in the ventral part of the pons or in the nerve itself.

Internuclear ophthalmoplegia is due to a tiny lesion in one medial longitudinal fasciculus, at a level between the nuclei of cranial nerves III and VI. The usual cause is multiple sclerosis (see Chap. 4). Interruption of the fibers going from the PPRF of the opposite side to the oculomotor nucleus of the same side causes inability to adduct the eye on the side of the lesion. There is also nystagmus of the abducting eye. The nystagmus is attributed to defective inhibition of the medial rectus of the abducting eye, caused by interruption of the axons of inhibitory internuclear neurons.

Paralysis of upward gaze is due to a lesion involving the "center for upward gaze" in the rostral part of the midbrain. Causes include pressure from a nearby tumor, such as one arising from the pineal gland, and isolated lesions of various diseases that produce widespread changes in the brain. The "center for downward gaze" is rarely put out of action.

Cranial Nerve Palsies

"Palsy" is an old word for paralysis, still used for disorders of single nerves or muscles. Abnormal eye movements can be difficult to diagnose. The first thing to do is to *determine which muscles are not working.* A single lesion causing disordered movement of both eyes must be in the central nervous system. If only one eye moves abnormally, a peripheral lesion is likely.

Defective alignment of the eyes is called **squint** or **strabismus.** Most often, squint is not due to paralysis or weakness of muscles. In such cases both eyes can move through a full range of positions. If one eye fails to converge, it will do so if the other eye is covered. This common condition is called a **concomitant squint.**

A malfunction of one or more of the extraocular muscles causes a **paralytic squint.** If paralysis is complete it is not usually difficult to decide which muscle or group of muscles is not working. When there is only weakness (paresis), however, the squint may be apparent only when the eye is attempting to move in the direction of action of the affected muscle. The first symptom is **diplopia** (double vision), which occurs because the central foveae of the two eyes cease to receive images of the same object. With time the brain suppresses the false image, so the symptom of diplopia disappears. The two golden rules in the diagnosis of diplopia are:

1. The separation of the images increases with the amount of movement in the direction of pull of the weak muscle (or muscles).
2. The false image (that is, the one in the abnormally moving eye) is displaced in the direction of action of the weak or paralyzed muscle(s).

If the patient cannot be sure which eye produces which image, the uncertainty can be resolved by placing colored glass in front of one eye.

With an **oculomotor nerve paralysis,** the eye is closed because the muscle that elevates the upper lid is denervated. If the lid is raised by hand, it is seen that the eye is deviated laterally by the unopposed action of the lateral rectus muscle. The pupil is widely dilated because the ciliary ganglion has been deprived of its preganglionic supply.

Trochlear nerve palsy causes diplopia when a person attempts to look downward and medially. This symptom is particularly disabling when one is walking down stairs. The condition can occur as a manifestation of a peripheral neuropathy (in diabetes mellitus, for example), and it is an occasional persistent complication of head injury.

Abducent nerve paralysis causes medial squint, because the lateral rectus is the only muscle that abducts the eyeball. Cranial nerve VI may be affected by a peripheral neuropathy, or the lateral rectus muscle itself may degenerate for an unknown reason.

All the extraocular muscles are sensitive to diseases that afflict skeletal muscle in a general way. **Myasthenia gravis** is a disease in which neuromuscular transmission is inhibited (see Chap. 13), thereby preventing the motor nerve from causing contraction of the muscle fibers it supplies. Weakness of the levator palpebrae superioris is often the first symptom, and weaknesses of the other extraocular muscles follow.

Sometimes cranial nerves III, IV, and VI are all involved in a single destructive lesion. This can be due to inflammation of unknown cause in the region of the superior orbital fissure or to compression of the nerves in the cavernous sinus (see Chap. 29).

Disorders of Visual Reflexes

Every medical examination includes testing the responses of the pupil to light and accommodation. In an unconscious patient, it is particularly important to take note of changes in the pupillary light reflex. The rationale for each of the following conditions should be obvious from the anatomy and physiology of the pathways involved.

A blind eye—no reflexes are elicited from it, although its iris is responsive to light shone into the other eye, if that is not blind.

A glass eye exhibits no responses to light shone in either eye. (This is an old favorite of clinical examiners of medical students.)

The Argyll Robertson pupil is an abnormally small pupil that constricts with accommodation but not when light is shone in the eye. Neuroanatomical teaching decrees that the lesion should be in the pretectal area, but this deduction is not always supported by post mortem observations. The iris itself is abnormal in many cases. This abnormal pupil is due to syphilis of the central nervous system. Douglas Argyll Robertson (1837–1909) was a Scottish ophthalmologist.

An *enlarged pupil that responds slowly to light* is occasionally seen in otherwise normal young (usually female) adults in the absence of any known disease.

The commonest abnormality of visual reflexes is impairment of the pupillary light reflex in a patient with deteriorating conscious level following a head injury. The usual cause is stretching of the oculomotor nerve over the free margin of the tentorium cerebelli as a result of pressure from a subdural hemorrhage (see Chapter 28).

Chapter 20

The Cranial Nerves

This chapter deals with cranial nerves **V, VII, IX, X, XI,** and **XII.** The sense of **taste,** served by three of these, is also covered here. The other cranial nerves have been discussed in other chapters. A table in Chapter 12 summarizes the principal functions of all the cranial nerves.

Nerve Components

A nerve component is a population of axons with a distinct function. The efferent components of cranial nerves have their cell-bodies in **nuclei of origin** in the brain stem. Afferent components have their cell-bodies in ganglia that correspond to the sensory ganglia of spinal nerves. The axonal branches that enter the brain stem end in **nuclei of termination.**

The following components are recognized in the cranial nerves:

1. *General somatic efferent.* Motor fibers supplying skeletal striated muscles derived from the myotomes (that is, the extraocular muscles and the muscles of the tongue).
2. *Special visceral (branchiomotor) efferent.* Motor fibers that supply striated skeletal muscles derived from the branchial arches—those that open and shut the mouth, or move parts of the face, larnyx, or pharynx.
3. *General visceral efferent.* These are preganglionic fibers; they terminate in the

parasympathetic ganglia of the head and in the enteric nervous system.
4. *Special visceral afferent.* Sensory fibers subserving smell and taste.
5. *General visceral afferent.* Sensory fibers from internal organs, including the heart, lungs, and alimentary canal (see Physiological Afferents, Chap. 27)
6. *General somatic afferent.* Ordinary sensations (touch, pain, proprioception) from skin, mucous membranes, muscles, and joints.
7. *Special somatic afferent.* These are the afferent fibers for special senses not associated with feeding: hearing, equilibration, and vision. (The optic nerve is not a nerve, but its sensory axons are formally included in this component, just as the optic nerve is formally numbered as the second cranial nerve.)

There is no named component that includes the efferent axons in the vetibulocochlear nerve (see Chaps. 16 and 17) or centrifugal fibers in the optic nerve that go from the brain to the retina (such fibers are well known in birds and have been demonstrated in some laboratory mammals). The reason for these omissions is that the classification of components was made up before the fibers efferent to receptors for the special senses were discovered. A term such as *"special somatic efferent"* might be appropriate for the centrifugal components of the second and eighth cranial nerves.

Table 20-1 lists the components of the cranial nerves, with nuclei of origin and termination. It is quite feasible to learn about the cranial nerves without understanding the components, but a summary of this kind helps to show that the body of information is not very large, and the functions of most of the nuclei are obvious from their names.

The positions of the cranial nerve nuclei are shown in Chapter 8 and are also indicated symbolically in the diagrams in this chapter.

Trigeminal Nerve

This nerve is named from its having three main branches, the **ophthalmic,** the **maxillary,** and the **mandibular** divisions. The nerve arises from the pons as a large sensory root and a small motor root. The somata of the primary sensory neurons are in the large **trigeminal ganglion,** which lies at the base of the skull ensheathed by dura. The ganglion is often called the "semilunar ganglion," or the "Gasserian ganglion" (after the 18th century Austrian anatomist, J.L. Gasser). The motor fibers are all distributed with the mandibular division. The other two divisions are entirely sensory.

The areas of the head supplied with sensory fibers by the divisions of the trigeminal nerve are illustrated in Figure 20-1.

The motor fibers of the trigeminal nerve supply the four muscles of chewing (masseter, temporalis, lateral pterygoid, medial pterygoid), three of the many muscles involved in swallowing (mylohyoid, anterior belly of digastric, and tensor veli palatini), and one of the small muscles of the middle ear (tensor tympani).

Table 20-1.   Components and Nuclei of the Human Cranial Nerves

Component	Nucleus	Nerve
General somatic efferent	Oculomotor nucleus	III
	Trochlear nucleus	IV
	Abducent nucleus	VI
	Hypoglossal nucleus	XII
Special visceral efferent	Trigeminal motor nucleus	V
	Facial motor nucleus	VII
	Nucleus ambiguus	IX, X, XI
	Accessory nucleus	XI
General visceral efferent	Edinger-Westphal nucleus	III
	Superior salivatory nucleus	VII
	Lacrimal nucleus	VII
	Inferior salivatory nucleus	IX
	Dorsal nucleus of vagus	X
	Nucleus ambiguus (part)	X
Special visceral afferent	Olfactory bulb (see Chap. 14)	I
	Rostral end of solitary nucleus (gustatory nucleus)	VII, IX, X
General visceral afferent	Solitary nucleus (caudal part)	IX, X
General somatic afferent	Trigeminal sensory nuclei	V, VII, IX, X
Special somatic afferent	Sites of termination of axons of optic tract (see Chap. 18)	II
	Cochlear and vestibular nuclei (Chaps. 16, 17)	VIII

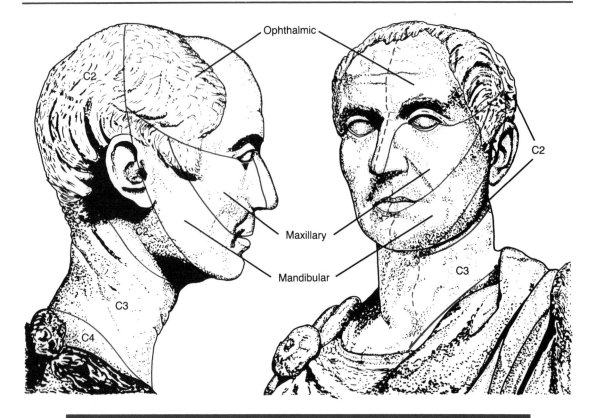

Figure 20-1 The areas supplied by the three divisions of the trigeminal nerve. Nearby cervical dermatomes are also shown (nerve C1 usually has no dorsal root). Dermatomes overlap (see Chap. 7), but the areas supplied by the divisions of the trigeminal nerve are sharply defined.

Central Connections (Fig. 20-2)

The sensory fibers passing centrally from the trigeminal ganglion are distributed to the different trigeminal sensory nuclei *in accordance with the modalities of sensation they subserve.* Fibers for pain and temperature sensation turn caudally in the spinal trigeminal tract and end in the **caudal part of the spinal trigeminal nucleus,** which is in the medulla and the first one or two cervical segments of the spinal cord. Fibers for general tactile sensation, including discriminative touch, end in the **pontine trigeminal nucleus** and

in the **rostral part of the spinal trigeminal nucleus.**

Fibers serving proprioception from the muscles of mastication, together with fibers receiving sensations of pressure from the sockets of the teeth, have a unique central connection. The primary sensory neurons are unipolar, but they are *not in the trigeminal ganglion.* Instead these neurons have their somata in the **mesencephalic trigeminal nucleus,** a slender column of cells that lies lateral to the aqueduct and to the most rostral part of the fourth ventricle. These are the only primary sensory neurons found in the central nervous system. The axons of the cells of the

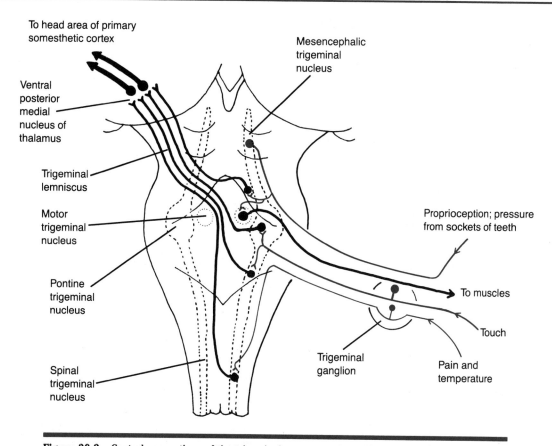

Figure 20-2 Central connections of the trigeminal nerve, together with the ascending somesthetic pathway for the head. The spinal trigeminal nucleus also receives the somatic sensory fibers of cranial nerves VII, IX, and X (see Figs. 20-3 and 20-4).

mesencephalic trigeminal nucleus descend in the mesencephalic trigeminal tract and bifurcate in the pons. The peripheral branches leave the brain stem in the trigeminal nerve; central branches go to the motor trigeminal nucleus, to the nearby pontine reticular formation, and to the pontine and spinal trigeminal nuclei.

The trigeminal sensory nuclei and connected cells in nearby areas of the reticular formation send **trigeminothalamic fibers** across the midline. After crossing, these fibers ascend as the trigeminal lemniscus and end in the **ventral posterior medial nucleus of the thalamus.**

This thalamic nucleus projects to the primary somatosensory cortex: the head area is at the lower end of the postcentral gyrus.

The motor axons originate in the **trigeminal motor nucleus,** which is in the pons, near the pontine trigeminal nucleus. The axons are distributed to the muscles already listed.

The motor trigeminal nucleus is controlled by descending pathways (see Chap. 23) from *both* cerebral hemispheres. Consequently, a destructive lesion in one hemisphere does not paralyze voluntary movements of the muscles of mastication. Ordinary chewing movements are largely controlled by local circuitry in the brain stem and cerebellum. Proprioception from the muscles and pressure sensations from the sockets of the teeth contribute importantly to the physiology of chewing.

Clinical Examination

Cutaneous sensation is tested in the area supplied by each division. The strength of the muscles of mastication can be assessed by palpating the masseter muscles when the teeth are clenched. The **jaw-jerk** is a reflex contraction of the mouth-closing muscles elicited by tapping downward on the point of the chin. This reflex tests the integrity of the proprioceptive and motor connections. The **corneal reflex** (blinking in response to touching the cornea with a wisp of cotton) tests sensory fibers of the ophthalmic division of V and the motor component of VII.

Disorders

Herpes zoster or **shingles** is a common condition in which there is a painful skin eruption in the area supplied by a sensory nerve root. The disease is caused by a virus (the same one that causes chickenpox) in primary sensory neurons. The manner of production of the inflamed skin may be similar to that of neurogenic inflammation (see Chap. 13). Herpes zoster can afflict any dermatome; it frequently occurs in the field of the ophthalmic division of V, causing pain in the eye and the appropriate area of skin, and sometimes giving rise to ulcers or scars of the cornea. Treatment is aimed mainly at relief of symptoms. Some *antiviral drugs,* including idoxuridine and vidarabine, are also used, especially in immunosuppressed patients.

  Trigeminal neuralgia, also called *tic douloureux,* produces brief but frequent stabs of excruciating pain in the territory of one or more divisions of the trigeminal nerve. The disease is caused in at least some patients, by a small unduly tortuous artery at the base of the brain bumping agaist and irritating the nerve. Surgical procedures to move the offending vessel out of the way are frequently successful. Other operations, such as destroying the ganglion, are now rarely needed. Most patients with trigeminal neuralgia are adequately relieved by *carbamazepine,* but it is not known why this drug, otherwise used to treat epilepsy, is effective.

Facial Nerve

The facial nerve has four functional components. Efferent fibers are motor and preganglionic parasympathetic. Sensory fibers are for taste and cutaneous sensation.

Anatomy

The nerve has two roots. The more medial **motor root,** is the larger. The other root, containing parasympathetic and sensory fibers, is called the **intermediate nerve** (*nervus intermedius*) because it is between the motor root and the vestibular nerve. Both roots of VII accompany the vestibular and cochlear nerves into the internal auditory meatus. The facial roots pass near the labyrinth and so reach the facial canal in the medial wall of the middle ear cavity. Here the two roots fuse, and the **geniculate ganglion,** containing somata of sensory neurons, is present. The name geniculate means "like a little knee' (Latin, *genu*), because at this point the nerve turns sharply in a posterior and inferior direction. After giving off four branches, the facial nerve leaves the skull through the stylomastoid foramen, curves forward beneath the external ear, and enters the parotid gland. There the nerve divides into branches that supply the muscles of the face and scalp.

  The following are the branches of the facial nerve, listed with their functions. The terminal parts of the sensory and parasympathetic fibers are distributed in branches of V, with which the branches of VII communicate through anastomotic nerve filaments.

1. *Greater petrosal nerve.* This leaves at the geniculate ganglion. It contains sensory fibers that innervate **taste buds on the soft palate** and preganglionic parasympathetic fibers that end in the **pterygopalatine ganglion** (also called "sphenopalatine"). The neurons in the ganglion supply the lacrimal gland, which secretes tears, and the small mucous glands of the nose.

2. *Nerve to stapedius.* This supplies the **stapedius muscle** of the middle ear. This muscle helps to protect the cochlea from loud noise by limiting the amplitude of vibration of the stapes.

3. *Chorda tympani.* This nerve leaves the facial canal just above the stylomastoid foramen. It runs anteriorly, crossing the inside surface of the tympanic membrane before passing through a tiny foramen into the infratemporal fossa. There the chorda tympani joins the lingual nerve, a branch of the mandibular division of the trigeminal. The taste fibers from the chorda tympani are distributed to the **anterior two thirds of the tongue.** The preganglionic parasympathetic fibers go to the **submandibular ganglion** (which is sometimes given the misleading name "submaxillary ganglion."). This ganglion supplies the submandibular and sublingual salivary glands and also the many tiny, unnamed salivary glands in the floor of the mouth.

4. *Cutaneous branch.* This filament leaves the nerve within the stylomastoid foramen and its fibers mingle with those of the auricular branch of the vagus nerve. Both nerves supply the posterior part of the external surface of the tympanic membrane, some of the skin of the exter-

nal meatus, part of the concha of the auricle, and an area just behind the external ear.

5. *Terminal branches.* These branches are the posterior auricular, temporal, zygomatic, buccal, mandibular, and cervical nerves. All carry motor fibers to the **muscles that move the scalp and the parts of the face.** The facial muscles are used for changing the expression, for keeping the lips and cheeks in position when chewing, and for closing the eyes.

Central Connections (Fig. 20-3)

The proximal branches of the axons of the sensory neurons of the geniculate ganglion go to two nuclei of termination in the medulla. Those for cutaneous sensation end in the **spinal trigeminal nucleus.** The axons for taste pass into the solitary tract and terminate in the **rostral end of the solitary nucleus.** This end of the solitary nucleus is also named the **gustatory nucleus,** because all primary afferent fibers for taste end there.

The preganglionic parasympathetic axons come from two groups of cells in the medulla. These are near the facial motor nucleus, but their exact positions in the human brain are not known. The **lacrimal nucleus** is the source of axons that end in the pterygopalatine ganglion. The **superior salivatory nucleus** sends axons to the submandibular ganglion.

The motor fibers constitute the largest component of the facial nerve. They arise from the **facial motor nucleus** in the caudal part of the pons and follow a curious curved course within the brain stem, looping dorsally around the abducent nucleus before turning ventrally.

The functions of the facial motor nucleus are controlled by descending pathways (see Chap. 23) from the cerebral hemispheres. The motor neurons supplying the lower half of the

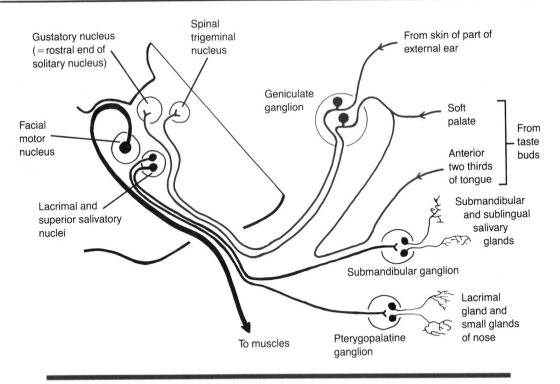

Figure 20-3   Components and connections of the facial nerve.

face resemble those of the limbs in being controlled by the contralateral cerebral hemisphere. *Motor neurons supplying the upper face (muscles that close the eye and elevate the eyebrows) are unusual in that they are controlled by both cerebral hemispheres.* This italicized statement embodies the principle whereby a facial weakness or paralysis is judged to be due to abnormality in the ipsilateral nerve or in the contralateral cerebral hemisphere.

Clinical Examination

Taste is not routinely tested, but it is worth remembering that sweet substances are detected at the tip of the tongue, an area where all the taste buds are supplied by axons from the facial nerve. Sour substances, because they are detected by the lateral edges of the tongue, may be used to lateralize a defect in taste sensation.

The **parasympathetic functions** of the facial nerve are not easy to test. Failure of secretion from the lacrimal gland can dry the cornea, with the risk of ulceration.

The **motor component** is the most important one from the clinical point of view. Weakness of the lower half of the face is sought by asking the patient to "show your teeth" and to blow out the cheeks with the mouth closed. Facial paresis causes weakness of the muscles that move the lips. Even without asking the patient to do anything it is usually possible to spot a facial paralysis by noting the absence of the crease that normally extends from the side of the nose to the angle of the mouth. The muscles of the upper half of the face are tested by asking the patient to close the eyes tightly against resistance from the physician's finger and thumb ("screw up you eyes and don't let me open them") and by observing the movements of the eyebrows and associated wrinkling of the forehead. Paralysis of the stapedius muscle can make ordinary sounds feel unpleasantly loud.

The face should also be watched for *involuntary changes in expression,* because this type of movement is usually spared by a lesion in the cerebral hemisphere that paralyzes voluntary movement of the lower half of the face.

The corneal reflex (also mentioned for cranial nerve V) has its efferent limb in the motor component of VII. The interneurons for the corneal reflex are in the medullary reticular formation, between the spinal trigeminal and the facial motor nuclei.

Disorders

Bell's palsy is the most common cause of facial paralysis. The disease is named after Charles Bell (1774–1842), a Scottish surgeon who was also one of the first people to recognize the separate functions of the dorsal and ventral spinal nerve roots. The paralysis is due to inflammatory swelling in the facial nerve, which causes compression within its bony canal. Loss of taste can usually be detected too. The disease may be due to a virus. There is no effective treatment, but most patients recover in less than 3 months.

The other common cause of facial paralysis or weakness is **a lesion in the contralateral cerebral hemisphere.** This affects *only the lower half of the face.* Often there is paralysis or weakness of other parts of the body at the same time. A facial paralysis of this kind *does not usually impair involuntary changes in*

facial expression. The neuroanatomical reason for this sparing is unknown. In Parkinson's disease (see Chap. 24), the face is expressionless because involuntary movements do not occur, although there is no impairment of voluntary facial movements.

Herpes zoster (described already as a disorder of the trigeminal nerve) can infect the geniculate ganglion, causing pain and inflammation in the external auditory meatus. This is a rare condition.

Hemifacial spasm consists of irregular facial twitchings, especially around the eye. It is sometimes due to irritation of the nerve by an abnormally situated branch of the anterior inferior cerebellar artery. An intracranial operation to move the vessel out of the way may be justifiable if the symptoms are distressing.

Glossopharyngeal Nerve

This nerve is sensory for the posterior third of the tongue, the pharynx, and the middle ear. It also supplies one small muscle and contains fibers with parasympathetic and visceral afferent functions.

The nerve is formed from rootlets rostral to those of the vagus. It leaves the cranial cavity through the jugular foreman, in company with cranial nerves X and XI and the internal jugular vein. There are two sensory **glossopharyngeal ganglia** (superior and inferior), near the level of the foramen. The preganglionic parasympathetic fibers end in the tiny **otic ganglion,** which supplies the parotid gland.

Central Connections (Fig. 20-4)

The sensory neurons have their somata in the glossopharyngeal ganglia. Those concerned

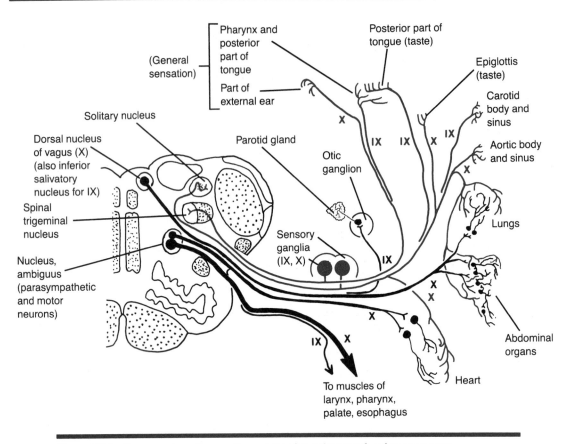

Figure 20-4   Components and connections of the glossopharyngeal and vagus nerves.

with general sensation project centrally to the **spinal trigeminal nucleus.** The taste fibers enter the solitary tract and terminate in the **gustatory nucleus,** which is the rostral pole of the solitary nucleus. The visceral afferent fibers in IX supply the carotid sinus and the carotid body. These are receptors for cardiovascular and respiratory reflexes. Their sensory neurons project centrally to the more **caudal parts of the solitary nucleus.**

Preganglionic parasympathetic axons in IX arise from the **inferior salivatory nucleus.** This is probably rostral to the dorsal nucleus of the vagus, but its exact position in man is un-known. Motor axons to the larynx and pharynx come from the **nucleus ambiguus.** Those in the glossopharyngeal nerve supply only the stylopharyngeus, one of the muscles used in swallowing.

Clinical Examination and Disorders

Sensation from the oropharynx can be tested by touching with a spatula. This usually elicits elevation of the soft plate (gag reflex), a movement of muscles supplied by the vagus nerve. Taste from the back of the tongue should be tested with a bitter substance.

Lesions affecting only the glossopharyngeal nerve are unlikely to be encountered. There is, however, a **glossopharnygeal neuralgia.** This disease is like trigeminal neuralgia, but the episodes of pain are felt in the throat, radiating to the ear. If carbamazepine is ineffective, the nerve can be transected in the neck.

Vagus Nerve

The name of this nerve means "wandering," the branches extend beyond the head and neck into the thorax and abdomen.

Anatomy

In the neck, the vagus supplies all the muscles of the larynx and pharynx (except the stylopharyngeus) and the striated muscle of the upper third of the esophagus. The preganglionic parasympathetic fibers end in small ganglia associated with the heart, the bronchi, and the alimentary tract as far along as the splenic flexure of the colon. The ganglia in the esophagus, stomach, and intestines constitute part of the enteric nervous system (see Chap. 27). Most of the sensory cell-bodies are in the **inferior vagal ganglion** (more often called the **nodose ganglion**) near the bifurcation of the carotid artery. The **superior vagal (jugular) ganglion** contains the somata of sensory fibers for a small area of the external ear, coextensive with the skin supplied by the facial nerve.

The rootlets of the vagus emerge between the inferior cerebellar peduncle and the olive and unite to form the nerve, which leaves the skull by way of the jugular foramen. Branches are given off in the neck, and there are several anastomosing branches in the thorax. The fibers reassemble as two nerves that pierce the diaphragm fore and aft of the esophagus. Branches enter the plexuses around the abdominal aorta and its branches, and are distributed to the viscera alongside the blood vessels.

Central Connections (see Fig. 20-4)

Four nuclei in the medulla are connected with the vagus nerve. The neurons concerned with general (somatic) sensation from the larynx, lower pharynx, esophagus, trachea, and part of the external ear send the central branches of their axons to the **spinal trigeminal nucleus.** (This nucleus receives all the sensory fibers from the skin and mucous membranes of the head; see Table 20-1.)

The neurons supplying the taste buds of the epiglottis project centrally to the **gustatory nucleus,** which is the rostral part of the solitary nucleus.

The **caudal parts of the solitary nucleus** receive the central branches of the axons of primary sensory neurons that deal with all the other visceral functions of the vagus nerve. Sensory signals come from the lungs, the heart, the chemo- and baro-receptors associated with the arch of the aorta, and the alimentary tract. The sensory information reaching the solitary nucleus is used in reflexes that control the functions of the viscera. Pain from internal organs follows other pathways (see Chap. 27).

The striated muscles of the larynx, pharynx, and esophagus are supplied by **motor neurons in the nucleus ambiguus.** This nucleus also contains some **preganglionic parasympathetic neurons** the axons of which end in ganglia associated with the heart. These mediate the slowing action of the vagus on the rate of the heart. The **dorsal nucleus of the vagus** contains all the other preganglionic autonomic neurons. Some of their axons end in small parasympathetic ganglia that supply the smooth muscle and glands of the respiratory passages. The largest numbers of axons from the dorsal nucleus end in the enteric nervous system. Activity of the vagus stimulates gastric and pancreatic secretion and promotes the movement of swallowed food from the esophagus to the descending colon.

Clinical Examination and Disorders

If a normal person says "aaah" with the mouth wide open, the soft palate and uvula can be seen to move upwards. If the pharyngeal muscles are paralyzed unilaterally, the uvula will deviate toward the normal side. Movement of the vocal cords can be checked with a laryngeal mirror, a technique requiring some skill and practice. Unilateral lesions do not affect visceral functions, and it is not feasible to test the sensory components of the vagus nerve.

Paralysis of the muscles supplied by the vagus may be due to a **destructive lesion involving the nucleus ambiguus** in the medulla. This can follow occlusion of the arterial supply to the lateral part of the medulla. Accompanying symptoms are due to involvement of the spinal trigeminal nucleus, the spinothalamic tract (see Chap. 15), and other nearby structures. A **lesion in a cerebral hemisphere** can paralyze the contralateral laryngeal and pharyngeal musculature. The lower half of the face, the tongue, and the limbs are also likely to be paralyzed or weak.

Transection of the vagus nerves below the diaphragm has often been done to reduce secretion of hydrochloric acid into the stomachs of patients with peptic ulcers. It is possible to cut only the branches to the fundus of the stomach, which contains most of the acid-secreting glands, thus sparing the branches that control emptying. Drugs such as cimetidine that selectively inhibit gastric acid secretion have greatly reduced the need for surgical treatment of peptic ulceration.

Accessory Nerve

Anatomy

Cranial nerve XI is something of an anatomical curiosity (see Fig. 8-1, Chap. 8). Some rootlets caudal to the vagal rootlets join to form the **cranial root** of the accessory nerve. Most of its axons are believed to come from the nucleus ambiguus. A larger **spinal root** is formed by rootlets arising from motor neurons in segments C1 to C5 or C6 of the spinal cord. These join to form a nerve (the spinal root of XI) that ascends through the foramen magnum and then becomes enclosed in the same sheath as the cranial root. The nerve thus formed is the complete accessory nerve. It leaves the cranium through the jugular foramen.

Once through the base of the skull, the accessory nerve immediately divides into an internal ramus and an external ramus (*Ramus* is Latin for "branch"). The **internal ramus,** which comprises the axons of the cranial root, joins the vagus nerve. The much larger **external ramus,** consisting of motor fibers from the cervical cord, descends into the neck and divides into branches that supply the **trapezius and sternocleidomastoid** (sternomastoid) muscles. These muscles also receive some motor fibers from the first two or three cervical nerves, and their proprioceptive innervation is from upper cervical dorsal roots.

Clinical Examination and Disorders

The functions of the cranial root of XI are inseparable from those of the motor fibers of the vagus. The trapezius and sternocleidomastoid muscles are easily tested by asking the patient respectively to "shrug your shoul-

ders" and "press your head against my hand."
By resisting these movements with his own
hands, the physician can easily assess the
functional states of the muscles supplied by
the spinal component of XI. It should be remembered that the sternocleidomastoid pulls
the head to the contralateral side.

Paralysis or weakness of the muscles supplied by the spinal root of XI usually is due
to a destructive **lesion in the contralateral cerebral hemisphere.** This paralysis is only a small
feature of the whole disorder.

Torticollis, or wryneck, is due to continuous
contraction (spasm) of the muscles of one side
of the neck, including those supplied by XI.
The usual cause is an injury, often apparently
trivial, to one of the cervical intervertebral
joints.

Hypoglossal Nerve

Anatomy (Fig. 20-5)

Cranial nerve XII supplies the **intrinsic and extrinsic muscles of the tongue.** The motor neurons
are in the **hypoglossal nucleus** in the lower part
of the medulla. Rootlets emerge between the
pyramid and the olive, and the complete
nerve leaves the cranium though its own foramen, the hypoglossal canal.

In the neck the hypoglossal nerve has anastomotic connections with the first two cervical
nerves. Experiments in animals indicate that
the muscle spindles in the tongue are innervated by the anastomotic nerves, by neurons
in the upper cervical spinal ganglia.

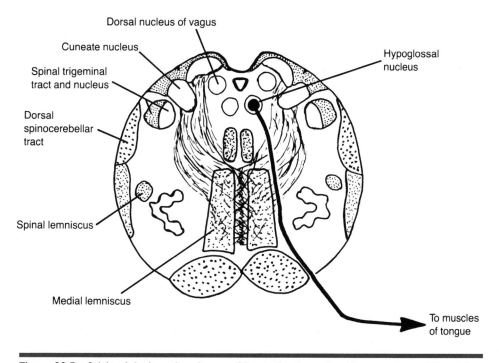

Figure 20-5 Origin of the hypoglossal nerve. (The section is at a level between those of Figs. 8-3
and 8-4.)

Clinical Examination and Disorders

Paralysis of the muscles supplied by XII prevents movements of the tongue on the afflicted side. Consequently, when the patient attempts to stick out his tongue the tip *deviates toward the side that is paralyzed or weak.* This is due to overaction of the muscles of the intact side.

The usual cause of hypoglossal paralysis is a **lesion in the contralateral cerebral hemisphere.** The axons passing ventrally from the hypoglossal nucleus are sometimes interrupted by a **lesion in the medial part of the medulla** (see Chap. 15, Fig. 15-4).

Pathway for Taste

It is appropriate to include the gustatory pathway in this chapter because the sense of taste enters the brain through cranial nerves VII, IX, and X.

Taste Buds

Most of the sense organs for taste are on the papillae of the tongue. Some also occur in the epithelia of the soft palate and the epiglottis. Each taste bud is an ellipsoidal nest of cells within the stratified squamous epithelium. Some cells in the bud are **gustatory cells** with cilia at their apical poles. Of the other cells, some fill in the spaces between the gustatory cells, and some are precursors of the mature cell-types. The cells of a taste bud live for only 1 or 2 weeks.

The cilia of the gustatory cells are in contact with the saliva, and they transduce chemical stimuli into a reduction of the cell's membrane potential. At its basal pole, each gustatory cell is contacted by a terminal branch of an axon. The contact resembles a chemical synapse, but the sensory cells are derived from ordinary epithelium, not neuroectoderm.

Four or five **primary tastes** are recognized: *Sweet, sour, bitter,* and *salty.* The taste buds most sensitive to these are on the tip, the lateral edges, the back of the tongue, and the middle of the tongue, respectively, although there is overlap. *Metallic* flavors, such as that of a licked copper coin, are perceived from all parts of the tongue. Sensation of each primary taste can be elicited from the human tongue by electrical stimulation if the electrode is fine enough to stimulate one taste bud at a time. Ordinary tastes are thought to result from mixed neural signals from at least four types of taste buds, integrated in the brain with the simultaneous activity of the olfactory system.

Taste buds provide an interesting example of a **trophic action** of peripheral nerves. If an area of the tongue is denervated, the taste buds disappear. Reinnervation results in the formation of new buds in the epithelium. The trophic maintenance of taste buds probably is mediated by a substance released from the ends of the sensory axons.

The Ascending Pathway

The neurons in the cranial nerve ganglia are unipolar. Their distal branches go to taste buds, and their central branches enter the **solitary tract** in the medulla, to end in the **gustatory nucleus,** which is the rostral pole of the solitary nucleus. The neurons in the gustatory nucleus have axons that go to the **parabrachial nucleus,** in the pontine reticular formation. The parabrachial nucleus projects to the **ventromedial basal nucleus of the thalamus.** This thalamic nucleus projects to the taste area of the cerebral cortex, which is behind (posterior to) the area of for general sensation from the mouth. The positions of the ascending fibers of the taste pathway in man are not known, and it is not known if the pathway crosses the midline.

Connections of the gustatory and parabrachial nuclei with the hypothalamus may be involved in autonomic reflex responses to taste, such as salivation, and in integrating the gustatory with the olfactory input to the brain.

Abnormalities of Taste

The only cause of loss of taste (**ageusia**) that is at all common is disease of the geniculate ganglion or of the facial nerve. The primary neurons or their axons are liable to be compressed by swelling in geniculate herpes zoster, Bell's palsy, or bacterial infection of the middle ear. A more common condition than ageusia is **anosmia** (see Chap. 14). An anosmic patient often describes the symptom as loss of taste, but the tongue can still detect sweet, sour, salty, and bitter substances.

Chapter 21

The Reticular Formation,

Consciousness,

and the Electroencephalogram

In Chapter 8, diagrams of transverse sections of the brain stem show well-defined tracts and nuclei. Much of the brain stem consists of nuclear groups that are not so easily delineated, together with interlacing small bundles of myelinated axons. The netlike appearance accounts for the name "reticular formation."

Reticular Nuclei and Their Connections

The neurons of the reticular formation are typically **isodendritic,** a term denoting that the dendrites have unusually long branches. These dendrites are spread out across the brain stem so that they can receive synaptic input from ascending and descending systems of fibers, including branches of the axons of other neurons of the reticular formation. Five groups of nuclei are recognized within the reticular formation (Fig. 21-1).

Precerebellar Reticular Nuclei

Three nuclei project to the cerebellar cortex. Afferent fibers reach the precerebellar reticular nuclei from the spinal cord, from the

vestibular nuclei, and from the cerebral cortex. These connections are presumed to collaborate with other cerebellar afferents in enabling the cerebellum to control and coordinate movements (see Chaps. 9 and 24).

Raphe Nuclei

The somata of these neurons are in the midline of the brain stem. The name "raphe" is from the Greek for "seam." The neurons are serotonergic (see Chap. 3, Table 3-1). Afferent fibers to the raphe nuclei come from the hypothalamus and from some parts of the forebrain. The axons of the serotonergic neurons are unmyelinated, greatly branched, and far-reaching. They extend caudally into the spinal cord and rostrally to the diencephalon and cerebral cortex. The extensive branching of the axons suggests that the raphe nuclei act in some general way, affecting many parts of the central nervous system simultaneously. Involvement in the level of consciousness and in depression or elation of mood are two functions that have been suggested.

A more definite function is known for some neurons in the raphe nuclei of the medulla. These cells have axons that descend in the

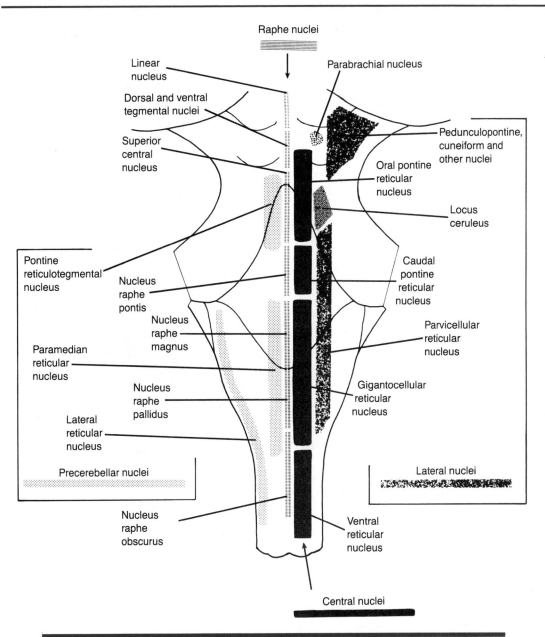

Figure 21-1 Approximate positions of the major nuclei of the reticular formation of the brain stem.

spinal cord and end in lamina II of the dorsal horn. Activity of these raphespinal fibers inhibits the upward transmission of impulses in the spinothalamic tract in response to otherwise painful stimuli (see Chap. 15).

Central Group of Reticular Nuclei

These nuclei in the medulla and pons contain neurons with large somata. Afferent fibers come from the spinal cord, from sensory nuclei of cranial nerves (especially V, VIII), from the superior colliculus, and from the cerebral cortex, notably the motor and premotor areas. The axons of the large neurons either ascend through the brain stem and terminate mainly in the intralaminar nuclei of the thalamus, or descend into the spinal cord in the reticulospinal tracts. Some of the neurons have axons that bifurcate into long ascending and descending branches. The neurons that project rostrally generally have their somata and dendrites caudal to those of the neurons that project caudally. This arrangement provides for synaptic interaction of collateral branches of axons with the dendrites of neurons that project in the opposite direction.

The **reticulothalamic** connections may be involved in sleep and arousal (see later in this chapter). The **reticulospinal** tracts constitute a major descending motor pathway.

Catecholamine Nuclei

Dopamine, noradrenaline, and adrenaline are **catecholamines.** Groups of neurons containing these substances are recognized by specific histochemical staining methods.

Neurons that make and store **noradrenaline** occur in several nuclei of the brain stem, the largest such population being the **locus ceruleus** (Latin, "blue place") in the rostral part of the pons. The noradrenergic neurons have long and richly branched unmyelinated axons that end in the gray matter of all parts of the brain and spinal cord. The fibers that go to the cerebellum and to the limbic system are mentioned in Chapters 9 and 25, respectively. The neurons of the locus ceruleus must influence many parts of the central nervous system simultaneously, and there is evidence that their noradrenaline acts as a neuromodulator (see Chap. 3), which inhibits or facilitates transmission across other chemical synapses.

Groups of neurons containing **dopamine** occur in the hypothalamus and midbrain. Some of the hypothalamic dopamine inhibits the release of prolactin, an adenohypophysial hormone (see Chap. 26). The dopamine-containing neurons of the midbrain are in the **substantia nigra** (projecting to the neostriatum; progressively destroyed in Parkinson's disease; see Chap. 24) and in the **ventral tegmental area** (which projects to the limbic system and hypothalamus). The dark color of the substantia nigra and the locus ceruleus is due to granules of melanin, a by-product of the synthesis of catecholamines. Groups of neurons that synthesize **adrenaline** have also been recognized in the medulla.

Lateral Group of Reticular Nuclei

Isodendritic neurons with small somata occur in the parvicellular reticular nucleus of the pons and medulla and in various nuclei in the midbrain. Axons afferent to the **parvicellular reticular nucleus** come from parietal areas of the cerebral cortex. The neurons of the parvicellular nucleus project medially to the central group of nuclei of the reticular formation.

The lateral group of reticular nuclei in the midbrain includes the following. The **pedunculopontine nucleus** is connected with the corpus striatum, indicating a role, albeit unknown, in movement. The **cuneiform nucleus** may direct stereotyped walking movements, at least in animals. The **parabrachial** nucleus has many connections. It is part of the pathway for taste, and may also be involved in the control of breathing. The name of the nucleus indicates its location medial to the superior cerebellar peduncle, which is sometimes called the *brachium conjunctivum* (Latin for "joining arm").

Various regions of the reticular formation are known to be essential for the control of such functions as respiration, heart rate, and blood pressure (see Chap. 27).

Arousal, Consciousness, and Sleep

Experiments with animals and clinical studies of people indicate that the integrity of the reticular formation is necessary for consciousness.

If the lower end of the medulla is transected, the animal must be artifically ventilated to be kept alive, because the motor neurons supplying the respiratory muscles have been separated from their controlling centers in the brain stem. Such an animal is called an *encéphale isolé* preparation (French for isolated brain). It is asleep most of the time, but can be aroused by noise or by touching the skin of the head. A decerebrate preparation, in which the midbrain has been transected, is called a *cerveau isolé* (isolated forebrain). It is unconscious and unrousable, although respiration occurs spontaneously. In order to produce permanent unconsciousness, a lesion must destroy the central nuclei of the reticular formation bilaterally in the upper pons or the midbrain. The same effect cannot be produced by large lesions in other parts of the brain stem. An animal with an electrode implanted in its reticular formation can be aroused from

normal sleep or from light general anesthesia by electrical stimulation.

These observations have led to the postulation that an **ascending reticular activating system** resides in the reticular formation, perhaps mainly in its central group of nuclei. The spinoreticular tracts and the equivalent pathways from sensory nuclei or cranial nerves *converge* on the reticular formation, which therefore receives afferent impulses concerned with many types of sensory stimuli from all parts of the body. The reticulothalamic pathway ends in the intralaminar nuclei of the thalamus. These project diffusely to large areas of the cerebral cortex.

Although the experiments cited above and the clinical conditions to be mentioned below support the idea that there is an ascending reticular activating system, this simple set of connections is certainly not enough to provide a complete explanation of the physiology of sleep. The main difficulty is that in normally sleeping animals and people there are intermittent periods in which the electroencephalogram (EEG) is quite similar to that of the awake subject. At such times there are *rapid eye movements,* so this type of sleep is known as **REM sleep.** It is often associated with dreaming. It has been hypothesized that memories are consolidated during REM sleep, and the suggestion has received some support from experiments in which animals undergoing training were deprived of REM sleep by administration of certain hypnotic (sleep-inducing) drugs, notably barbiturates.

It is not easy to reconcile the periodic episodes of REM sleep with an ascending reticular activating system driven largely by nonspecific sensory signals. There is much evidence for increased activity of neurons including those of the serotonergic raphe nuclei, in sleep. Another observation that does not fit in is the induction of sleep in animals by electrical stimulation of the posterior hypothalamus.

Electroencephalography

Activity in the cerebral cortex is recorded by amplifying electrical signals detected on the surface of the scalp. The fluctuations of voltage with time are plotted as the **electroencephalogram (EEG);** traces are made simultaneously from several points on both sides of the head. More exact localization is possible by recording directly from the exposed cortical surface (*electrocorticography*) in experimental animals or neurosurgical patients.

The fluctuations of voltage in the EEG are caused by the summed currents that result from postsynaptic potentials in dendrites. These small currents due to EPSPs and IPSPs (see Chap. 3) can spread over greater distances than the briefer currents caused by action potentials in axons. The EEG is probably due largely to activity of the large dendrites of the cortical pyramidal neurons (Chap. 22).

The normal EEG includes various wave forms (Fig. 21-2). All the waves have frequencies much lower than the rates of firing of action potentials of individual neurons. The EEG therefore represents summed, roughly synchronous changes in the dendrites of large numbers of neurons. The cause of the synchronization is the existence of inhibitory interneurons in the thalamus. These cells are excited by collateral branches of the axons of the thalamocortical projection neurons. Thus when a thalamocortical neuron discharges at a high frequency, it causes excitation of (a) the dendrites of cortical neurons, and (b) inhibitory thalamic interneurons. Each thalamic interneuron inhibits several thalamocortical projection neurons, thereby reducing their rates of discharge. The thalamocortical

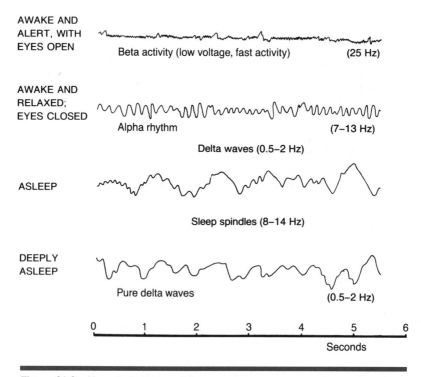

Figure 21-2   Normal electroencephalograms.

projection cells also receive excitatory synapses. Activation of the thalamocortical neurons will overcome the inhibitory effect of the interneurons, so that the cortex receives faster volleys of presynaptic action potentials. The frequency of the slower summed dendritic potentials will then increase. Excitation of thalamocortical projection neurons occurs in the alert condition. Accordingly, the EEG of the fully awake brain displays fast, asynchronous waves. Regular, slower waves are seen with a relaxed subject whose eyes are closed. Even slower rhythms, also attributable to interplay between cortex and thalamus, are recorded in sleep (Fig. 21-2).

Abnormalities in the EEG are associated with **epilepsy** (see Chap. 22), for which electroencephalography is a valuable diagnostic technique. A completely flat EEG is a widely accepted criterion of **death** of the cerebral cortex.

Abnormal Unconsciousness

Sleep is a normal state, but loss of consciousness can also be due to diseases. The major disorders of consciousness are **stupor,** from which the patient can be roused, but not fully, and **coma,** from which the patient cannot be roused. The many causes of stupor and coma fall into main groups: Diseases of the brain itself and abnormalities of general metabolism that affect the brain. A few examples follow.

The idea of an ascending reticular activating system fits in rather well with observations of diseases of the brain stem. Thus bilateral destruction of the medial parts of the reticular formation causes coma only if the lesion is at or rostral to midpontine level. **Infarction or hemorrhage in the pons** can cause coma in this way. Recovery sometimes occurs, presumably through the utilization of spared connections. A large bilateral lesion in the ventral part of the pons causes loss of all voluntary movements except those of the eyes, but the ascending sensory pathways and the reticular formation are intact, so the unfortunate patient is fully alert. This condition is called the **"locked in syndrome."** (*Syndrome* is a much misused word that means a collection of symptoms and signs that occur together, but need not always be caused by the same disease.)

A large space-occupying lesion in or near the cerebral hemispheres can cause **pressure on the brain stem** by an indirect mechanism described in Chapter 28, so causing deterioration of consciousness. The transient stupor or coma that follows an **epileptic seizure** is perhaps attributable to temporary failure of the ascending reticular activating system. **Concussion** that follows a head injury consists of impaired consciousness associated with loss of memory, from a short time before the injury until the patient is alert again. The abnormal neurophysiology causing the symptoms of concussion is not understood.

Metabolic causes of stupor and coma, such as hypoglycemia and renal failure, are outside the scope of this book.

Chapter 22

The Cerebral Cortex

In this chapter the functions of different parts of the cerebral cortex are discussed and related to the clinical consequences of destructive lesions. Epilepsy, the most common disease of the nervous system, is briefly reviewed too, because some of its manifestations are mediated by the cortex.

In Chapter 12 it is pointed out that in the tubular telencephalon of an amphibian or a reptile the pallium forms the dorsal wall of the lateral ventricle, separating the septum from the corpus striatum. In mammals the forebrain has a less obviously tubular structure and the pallium forms a layer, the cerebral cortex, that covers most of the outside surface of the cerebral hemisphere. The human cerebral cortex is folded into many convolutions, enclosing a large volume of subcortical white matter. The latter includes the corpus callosum, which interconnects the left and right cortices and forms the roofs of the lateral ventricles. Growth of the ventricular system causes what would otherwise be the medial edge of the pallium to lie next to the temporal horn of the lateral ventricle.

In reptiles three parts of the pallium are recognized: The **archipallium** is next to the septum, the **paleopallium** is next to the corpus striatum, and the **neopallium** (not present in fishes or amphibians) is in between. These relations also exist in the human cerebral cortex. Thus the **archicortex** constituting the hippocampal formation is medial to the temporal horn of the lateral ventricle and has a tenuous prolongation, the indusium griseum, that extends over the top of the corpus callosum to the septal area. The **paleocortex,** receiving the olfactory tract, is next to a part of the corpus striatum, the tail of the caudate nucleus. The **neocortex** accounts for most of the human pallium; it abuts the paleocortex on the inferior (ventral) surface of the temporal lobe (Fig. 22-1).

Regional Variation in Structure

It is possible to subdivide the cerebral cortex into **numbered areas** based on variations in histological structure. The most used set of numbers is that introduced by K. Brodmann (1868–1918), a German psychiatrist who studied cortical histology. In several places Brodmann's numbers correspond to functional areas defined by clinical studies, but there are more histologically recognized areas than there are functionally understood ones.

Figure 22-2 is provided for reference. It shows some of Brodmann's numbers. See also Figure 11-1 in Chapter 11 for names of sulci and gyri.

The archicortex and paleocortex are three-layered. The layers, starting at the surface, are: *Molecular layer* consisting largely of synapses, *pyramidal cell layer,* containing the large principal cells, and a *polymorphic*

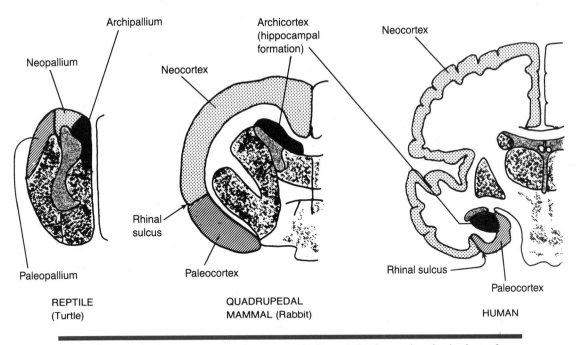

Figure 22-1   Transverse sections through the rostral telencephalon in a series of animals, to show the positions and relative sizes of the archi-, paleo-, and neocortex. The cavity of the lateral ventricle is colored. (Compare with Fig. 12-6.) In the human brain, the growth of the neocortex and of the corpus callosum produces the temporal lobe, containing an extension of the lateral ventricle and the archicortex of the hippocampal formation.

cell layer, containing principal cells and interneurons. Three-layered cortex is also called **allocortex.** The extensive neocortex, also called **isocortex,** has six layers: (1) *Molecular layer* (mainly synapses); (2) *external granular layer* (mostly interneurons); (3) *external pyramidal layer;* (4) *internal granular layer;* (5) *internal pyramidal layer;* and (6) *multiform layer* (containing principal cells of varied shape).

The thicknesses of the layers differ regionally over the cerebral cortex. In the motor areas of the frontal lobe, for example, the granular layers are inconspicuous (agranular cortex), whereas in the primary sensory areas layers two and four are particularly thick and there are not many pyramidal cells (granular cortex). The six layers are distinct in the remainder of the neocortex, but in the parahippocampal gyrus both granular layers are external to both pyramidal layers. The cingulate gyrus consists of cortex that is six-layered but is said to be intermediate between isocortex and allocortex.

Functional Areas and Their Disorders

The paleocortex, which is the area of termination of the olfactory tract, was discussed in Chapter 14. The archicortex of the hippocampal formation is a major part of the limbic system (see Chap. 25). The functionally dif-

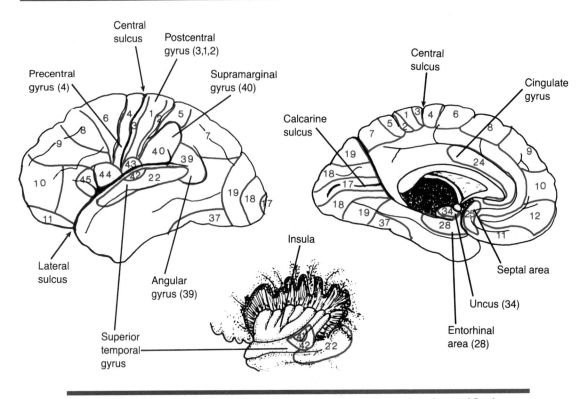

Figure 22-2   Areas of the human cerebral cortex numbered according to the scheme of Brodmann. Some anatomical names are also shown.

ferent regions of the neocortex will be reviewed here.

Primary Sensory Areas

The **primary somesthetic area** receives afferent fibers from the ventral posterior nucleus of the thalamus, which receives ascending sensory pathways from the contralateral skin and muscles. Somatotopic representation in the sensory pathways ensures that each part of the surface of the body sends its sensory signals to a particular region within the primary somaesthetic area. The half-body is represented as being upside down and has disproportionately large areas of cortex for the hands and face. A somatotopically organized

second sensory area is present in the roof of the lateral sulcus, but its functional significance is not understood.

Cortical areas for **vestibular sensation** and for **taste** are near the somaesthetic head area. Signals from vestibular receptors are also sent to the temporal lobe (see Chap. 17).

The **primary auditory area** faces upward into the lateral sulcus. It is tonotopically organized and receives projections concerned with both ears. Afferent fibers come from the medial geniculate body.

The **primary visual cortex** is in and around the calcarine sulcus, extending onto the gyri above and below. The retinotopic projection to this area is described in Chapter 18. Afferent fibers come from the lateral geniculate body.

The primary sensory areas are connected by subcortical association fibers with the appropriate sensory association areas.

Sensory Association Areas

A primary sensory area receives information about the events reported by the appropriate ascending pathway, but it cannot recognize or appreciate the importance of the sensation. The higher functions of recognition and use of sensory data reside in association cortex. These large areas, not always clearly defined, are adjacent to the primary sensory areas. Thus the association cortex for general somatic sensation is posterior to the postcentral gyrus. The association area for vision occupies much of the occipital lobe, together with the inferolateral cortex of the temporal lobe. The auditory association cortex is posterior to the primary area on the superior and lateral surfaces of the superior temporal gyrus. The olfactory association area is the entorhinal cortex and the more posterior parts of the parahippocampal gyrus.

In addition to association fibers from the primary sensory areas, the sensory association areas receive projection fibers from several thalamic nuclei (see Chap. 10).

A large lesion in an association area causes difficulty with recognition of words, objects, and things that are seen or felt. This recognition of significance is called *gnosis* (Greek for "knowledge"). Disorders of the sensory association areas cause various kinds of **agnosia.** An agnosia may be visual, auditory, or tactile. The most common form of tactile agnosia is **astereognosis,** the inability to identify objects felt with the hand. The word astereognosis is also commonly used for inability to discern differences in shape and texture with the fingers. This symptom is due to a lesion involving the hand area of the contra-lateral primary somaesthetic cortex. It is really a sensory deficit rather than an agnosia.

Language Areas

Cortical areas concerned with verbal and written communication are in the temporal, parietal, and frontal lobes. *These areas are concerned with language in only one of the hemispheres, usually the left.* The temporoparietal area is the **receptive language area,** which includes parts of the superior temporal, angular, and supramarginal gyri. Its integrity is necessary for the recognition of spoken and written words. It is also called Wernicke's area, after Carl Wernicke (1848–1905), a German clinical neurologist. The receptive language area receives afferent fibers from the auditory and visual association areas of both hemispheres. It is also connected with the expressive language area in the left frontal lobe. The **expressive language area** is often called Broca's area. Paul Broca (1824–1880), a French physician, was one of the first people to detect functional differences between the left and right cerebral hemispheres. The integrity of Broca's area is necessary for speech to communicate ideas formulated by the mind. The supplementary motor area is also essential for speech.

Disordered speech due to loss of function of cortical language areas is called **dysphasia,** or **aphasia** if the condition is very severe. These works have Greek roots meaning difficulty with or loss of speech.

Receptive aphasia results from damage to Wernicke's receptive language area. The patient cannot understand the meaning of words and usually cannot think of the names of objects or people.

Expressive aphasia is due to loss of function of Broca's expressive speech area. Although the patient knows what he wants to say, he cannot produce sensible words either in speech or in writing.

Conduction aphasia is due to severance of the subcortical association fibers that connect the receptive language area with the expressive speech area. Comprehension is not impaired, but the patient says incorrect words frequently and there is difficulty with repetition and with reading aloud.

Conditions related to aphasia include **agraphia** (inability to write), which commonly accompanies other types of aphasia. **Alexia** is inability to understand written language, and it commonly accompanies receptive aphasia. In *pure alexia* there is no difficulty in understanding spoken words. The lesion, near the occipital horn of the left lateral ventricle, interrupts the callosal fibers joining the visual association areas and also the association fibers connecting the left visual association area with the receptive speech area.

Mutism is complete loss of the power of speech. It occurs with lesions involving both supplementary motor areas. More common causes are psychiatric diseases with no anatomical abnormality of the brain. Cortical disorders of speech must not be confused with defective functioning of the muscles of the mouth, tongue, and larynx, which may be due to lesions affecting the cranial nerves or the cerebellum.

Motor Areas

Four cortical areas have motor functions. These are regions from which movements are elicted by electrical stimulation.

The **primary motor area** is Brodmann's area 4, on the precentral gyrus. On this strip of cortex, the opposite half of the body is represented upside down, in a pattern similar to that of the primary somaesthetic area. Electrical stimulation causes simple, purposeless movements due to concerted contraction of groups of muscles, with relaxation of their antagonists.

A small lesion in the primary motor area causes paralysis or weakness of the movements appropriate to the cortical site destroyed. The affected muscles are not spastic (see Chap. 23), and recovery may ensue because the surrounding areas of cortex can take over the function of the small lost part.

The **supplementary motor area** is on the medial surface of the hemisphere, anterior to the foot and lower leg zones of the primary motor area. Both sides of the body are represented in both supplementary motor areas. Electrical stimulation causes bilateral movement.

A unilateral destructive lesion causes difficulty in initiating movements on the contralateral side and impairment of activities that require the use of both hands together. Bilateral lesions cause greater loss of spontaneous movement, together with mutism.

The **premotor cortex** is anterior to the precentral gyrus on the lateral aspect of the hemisphere, in Brodmann's area 6. The frontal eye field in area 8 is nearby (see Chap. 19).

Destructive lesions in the premotor cortex cause weakness of the muscles that move the limbs at the shoulder and hip joints.

The **second motor area** is coextensive with the second sensory area in the roof of the lateral sulcus, inferior (ventral) to the primary motor and sensory areas. Movements and sensations are elicited bilaterally by electrical stimulation of this area, which is not shown in Fig. 22-3, but no functional defects have been attributed to lesions there.

The motor areas receive abundant association fibers from the sensory areas and ascending fibers from the ventral lateral nucleus of the thalamus. The pyramidal cells of the motor cortical areas project to the spinal cord, the pontine nuclei, the reticular formation, and the corpus striatum.

Apraxia is clumsiness of movement due to cerebral cortical dysfunction. A lesion in the

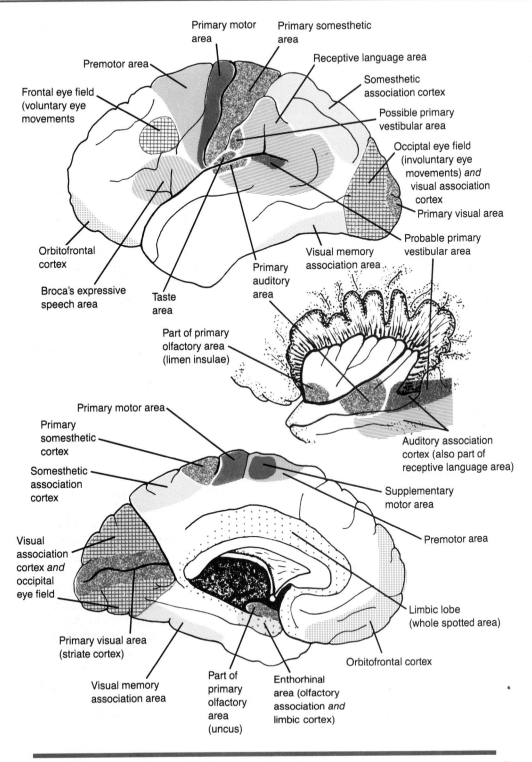

Figure 22-3 Functional areas of the human cerebral cortex.

left parietal lobe is often responsible for bilateral apraxia associated with a receptive aphasia. Right-sided apraxia results from subcortical lesions that severe connections between the left parietal and frontal lobes, and left-sided apraxia can be due to transection of those fibers of the corpus callosum that connect the parietal lobes. A form of apraxia manifest as inability to dress and undress is attributed to damage in the right parietal lobe.

Other Areas

Large areas of the frontal, parietal, temporal, and insular lobes are not primary sensory, sensory association, language, or motor areas. Nonetheless, all such parts of the cortex have their own connections and functions, but these cannot always be deduced confidently from the effects of electrical stimulation or of destructive lesions.

The **prefrontal cortex** covers the frontal lobe rostral (anterior) to areas 6 and 8, including the orbital (inferior) surface. In addition to association fibers connecting with all other areas of the cerebral cortex, the prefrontal lobe is connected with the amygdala and with the large mediodorsal nucleus of the thalamus. The prefrontal cortex is used in the appreciation and understanding of *time,* and is essential for normal *affect* (or feelings).

Destructive lesions of the prefrontal cortex, or of its subcortical white matter, must be bilateral to have any effect. The most prominent changes are loss of the ability to predict the consequences of things that are said or done and reduced elation or sadness in response to events that would normally provoke these feelings. Loss of function of the orbital cortex may be especially involved in producing these abnormalities, which can include irresponsible or inconsiderate social behavior. **Prefrontal leukotomy** (sometimes called "lobotomy") is surgical transection of white matter in the ventral part of the frontal lobe, cutting connections of the orbital cortex with the thalamus and amygdala. The operation was once fashionable for the treatment of depression and other abnormal mental states that were unresponsive to other forms of treatment. Leukotomy can also relieve severe pain: The painfulness is unchanged, but the patient is no longer bothered by it.

In the **parietal lobe** of the hemisphere that does not accomodate the language area (usually the right), the equivalent region has other functions. The most conspicuous of these is the recognition and interpretation of shapes and textures, especially in three dimensions and when the information cannot easily be put into words, as in the case of the contours of a face. The posterior part of the parietal lobe of the nonlinguistic hemisphere is also involved, in a general way, in the appreciation of the existence of the opposite side of the body and of the outside world.

A patient with a destructive lesion in the superior part of the right parietal lobe may deny the presence of the left arm and leg and may ignore all objects in the left visual field. This strange condition is called **neglect.** Another change in patients with lesions in the right parietal lobe is loss of the ability to appreciate music, although auditory function is unimpaired.

The cortex of the **limbic system** includes the parahippocampal gyrus, the cingulate gyrus, and the hippocampal formation. These areas are involved in memory, in the higher control of the autonomic nervous system, and perhaps in the less easily defined mental activities of motivation and emotion.

Large areas of the **neocortex of the temporal lobe** are evidently involved in long-term memory. Electrical stimulation evokes a variety of mental images. These include *déjà vu* (French for "already seen"), a feeling of familiarity with one's surroundings, and *jamais vu* ("never seen"), a feeling of unnatural strangeness. There may also be auditory hallucinations of formed speech and visual hallucinations of scenes remembered from the past. These effects of stimulation indicate that the temporal neocortex is involved in some way in the storage and recall of memories. This cortex is close to auditory and visual association areas and to the language areas, a position perhaps well suited to the integration of edited information derived from multiple sensory systems.

Functions of the Commissures

The corpus callosum consists of pyramidal cell axons that cross the midline and terminate in the contralateral cerebral cortex. All areas of the neocortex are symmetrically connected by callosal fibers, *except*

1. The primary somaesthetic area, other than the cortex receiving projections from those parts of the head, neck, and trunk that are near the midline.
2. Regions of the primary visual cortex other than those receiving information from the overlapping vertical strip common to the visual fields of both eyes.
3. Certain parts of the temporal lobes, which are interconnected by the anterior commissure.

The sensory association areas are connected by particularly large numbers of commissural fibers.

Normally any information delivered to the cortex of one cerebral hemisphere is immediately shared with the other hemisphere as a result of activity of the neurons that give rise to commissural axons. All memory is thus stored bilaterally. For many years the corpus callosum was thought to be unimportant despite its large size, because a few people with no histories of neurological disease were found to have congenital absence of the commissure. More careful testing, however, reveals deficits that would be expected to result from disconnection of the hemispheres. The first thorough studies were made by Roger W. Sperry of the California Institute of Technology, Pasadena. He investigated patients with epilepsy (see later in this chapter) in whom the corpus callosum had been surgically transected to restrict the seizures to one side of the brain. The operation is called commissurotomy.

Postoperatively the patient is unable to name an object placed unseen in the left hand. This is because the identification of the object made by the sensory association area of the right cerebral cortex cannot be communicated to the left cortex, where the areas concerned with names and speech are located. The study of patients after commissurotomy also reveals the role of the right cerebral hemisphere in the appreciation of three-dimensional shapes. There is difficulty in distinguishing between similarly shaped objects held unseen in the left hand. Sperry, who has also done important research in developmental neurobiology, received half of the Nobel prize for Physiology or Medicine in 1981. The other half was shared by Hubel and Wiesel (see Chap. 18).

A partial commissurotomy occurs if there is obstruction of the artery that supplies the splenium of the corpus callosum. The splenium connects the visual association areas of the occipital lobes. Destruction of the splenium prevents the transfer of information from the right occipital cortex to the language areas of the left side. Consequently the patient is unable to name things seen only in the left visual field and may be unable to read the words on the left side of a page.

Epilepsy

Epilepsy is any condition in which, from time to time, the brain is afflicted with outbreaks of uncontrolled neuronal activity. These outbreaks usually cause loss of consciousness and abnormal movements. An epileptic episode of any kind is a **seizure.** If there are convulsive movements, it is often called a **fit.** An **aura** is a conscious feeling that some patients experience immediately before losing consciousness.

The commonest kind of epilepsy in adults is the **generalized form,** variously known as "central," "centrencephalic," "cryptogenic," or "idiopathic" epilepsy. The multitude of names attests to the unknown cause of the disease. It is believed that the neuronal discharges that initiate the seizures originate in the diencephalon or brain stem. The seizures are of the *grand mal* (French for "great evil") type. All the muscles contract for a few seconds in the tonic phase, and then there are intermittent contractions and relaxation in the clonic phase. Often there is no aura. The EEG of a patient with this type of epilepsy may show abnormally large low-frequency waves or intermittent bursts of high-voltage spikes (Fig. 22-4).

Electroconvulsive therapy (ECT) is the production of a *grand mal* seizure by applying an electric shock to the head. The actual fit is prevented by administration of suxamethonium and an anesthetic. ECT can bring about rapid relief from depression, but nobody knows why.

Petit mal epilepsy ("little evil") occurs in children and often disappears with maturity. Each seizure is a loss of consciousness lasting less than 1 second. The patient does not usually fall. Occasionally there is slight muscular twitching. The EEG shows characteristic spike-and-wave formations between attacks. This EEG pattern suggests, by analogy with results of experiments with animals, that *petit mal* attacks begin with abnormal neuronal discharges in the thalamus.

The rarest type of epilepsy is the best understood. This is **focal epilepsy,** in which the seizure begins at an identified site in the brain. This spot, the epileptogenic **focus,** is often an area of gliosis due to an old injury, or it may be an abscess or a tumor. The aura of a focal seizure is attributable to stimulation in the region of the focus. The stimulated area then expands from this site, producing progressive effects that may develop into a generalized *grand mal* attack or may be confined to one lobe or hemisphere. The classical type of focal seizure is *Jacksonian epilepsy,* named after John Hughlings Jackson (1835–1911), an English clinical neurologist who made important discoveries about the localization of functions

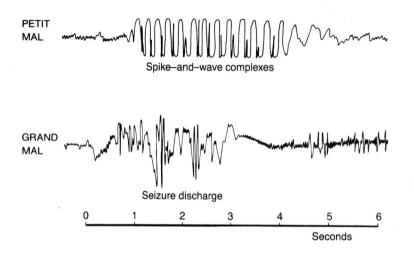

PETIT MAL

Spike–and–wave complexes

GRAND MAL

Seizure discharge

0   1   2   3   4   5   6

Seconds

Figure 22-4 Abnormal electroencephalograms showing records typically found in two common forms of epilepsy.

in the brain. A Jacksonian attack begins as small movements in part of one limb, such as a finger, then spreads gradually to the remainder of the limb, to the other muscles of the same side of the body, and finally to the contralateral side. The focus is in the primary motor area, and the progress of the movements illustrates the positions on the precentral gyrus that represent the different groups of muscles.

Temporal lobe epilepsy is the commonest condition associated with partial seizures. One cause is gliosis following pressure of the uncus on the tentorium cerebelli when the head is squeezed during birth. A temporal lobe seizure typically produces hallucinations of nasty but unidentifiable smells, *déjà vu,* feelings of fear or anxiety, and autonomic manifestations such as sweating, tachycardia (fast heart rate), and peculiar abdominal sensations. Rarely there may be irrational speech or behavior, which the patient does not remember afterwards. The temporal lobe does not greatly influence an ordinary EEG recording. It is sometimes considered justifiable to introduce needle electrodes alongside the sphenoid bone to seek abnormalities of the ventral surface of the temporal lobe.

Two abnormal EEG tracings are shown in Figure 22-4. The student should compare these with the normal records in Chapter 21 (see Fig. 21-2).

Anticonvulsant drugs are available for the treatment of the various types of epilepsy. They reduce the frequency and severity of the attacks. With focal epilepsy it is sometimes feasible to excise the focus surgically and cure the condition.

Chapter 23

Descending Pathways Involved in the Control of Movement

Movements are made by striated skeletal muscles, which contract in response to impulses transmitted by the motor neurons that supply them. Each motor neuron receives many excitatory and inhibitory synapses. Some of these operate reflexes at segmental levels (see Chap. 7). Other synapses mediate the effects of tracts that arise at higher levels of the neuraxis. Most descending axons end on interneurons, but some fibers, from the cerebral cortex and from the vestibular nuclei, synapse directly with motor neurons.

Modulation of Spinal Reflexes

The most important reflexes regulating contraction are those originating in the muscle spindles and the neurotendinous spindles. The muscle spindle responds to relative differences in *length* of the spindle and the surrounding ordinary (extrafusal) muscle fibers. Neurotendinous spindles respond to the amount of *tension* in the muscle; their activity causes inhibition of the motor neurons supplying the muscle, with excitation of the neurons supplying antagonistic muscles. The net result of unmodified spinal reflex activity is a state of sustained contraction of all the muscles. Normally this state is prevented by

the descending tracts, which have an overall inhibitory effect on the spinal reflexes.

If the spinal cord is transected, the muscles supplied by segments below the level of the transection are at first relaxed, or flaccid, and even the stretch and flexor reflexes are suppressed. This condition, called **spinal shock,** may be due to excessive activity of spinal inhibitory interneurons. After a few days the muscles develop a state of continuous weak contraction and are said to be **spastic.** The stretch and flexor reflexes are now exaggerated, so that an attempt to move any joint is resisted by muscular contraction, and a noxious stimulus evokes an inappropriately large withdrawal movement. The resistance to movement of a joint is of the "clasp knife" type: There is sudden relaxation of the resisting muscles when the amount of applied force is gradually increased. The relaxation is attributed to the reflex engendered by pulling on the neurotendinous spindles. Spastic paralysis also occurs with destructive lesions that involve the descending motor pathways in the cerebral hemisphere or brain stem.

Pyramidal System

The pyramidal system consists of the pyramidal tract (**corticospinal fibers**) and the equivalent **corticobulbar fibers** that end in or near the motor nuclei of cranial nerves V, VII, IX, X, XI, and XII.

Corticospinal and corticobulbar fibers are the axons of neurons in a large area of the cortex of the frontal and parietal lobes. This area includes the primary motor, premotor, supplementary motor, second motor, and primary somaesthetic areas. The axons pass in the posterior limb of the **internal capsule.** Their exact position there is still disputed. The fibers then pass caudally to become the middle part of the **basis pedunculi** of the midbrain. In the pons the descending fibers of the pyramidal system break up into small bundles among the transversely oriented pontocerebellar fibers, before reuniting to form the pyramid on the ventral surface on the medulla. At the caudal end of the medulla, most of the corticospinal axons cross the midline in the **decussation of the pyramids** and continue down the spinal cord in the lateral funiculus as the **lateral corticospinal tract.** A small proportion of corticospinal fibers do not cross in the pyramidal decussation. These uncrossed fibers form the ventral corticospinal tract in the ventral funiculus of the cord. Axons of the ventral corticospinal tract cross the midline at various segmental levels before entering the ventral horn of the spinal gray matter. Most corticospinal axons end on interneurons in lamina VII. Many end in the dorsal horn (see Chap. 15), and a few end on the dendrites and somata of the motor neurons in lamina IX.

Although the pyramidal tract is anatomically conspicuous, its functions are incompletely understood. The corticospinal fibers can be selectively transected only in the medulla or in the middle part of the basis pedunculi. Restricted lesions in these sites are described, although their occurrence is very rare, in man. Such lesions have also been studied experimentally in monkeys. The initial effect is flaccid paralysis of the contralateral musculature. With time the paralysis recovers and the residual disability is an inability to carry out movements of the hand that demand simultaneous use of more than one finger. The simplest conclusion from such observations is that normally the corticospinal fibers mediate much of the ordinary control of the muscles by the highest levels of the brain, but that the functions of this pathway can be usurped by other descending tracts for most purposes other than the performance of skilled manual tasks.

Reticulospinal Tracts

Reticulospinal fibers are the axons of neurons in the central nuclei of the reticular formation of the pons and medulla (Fig. 23-1). The **pontine reticulospinal tract,** in the ventral funiculus of the cord, originates ipsilaterally but terminates bilaterally. The more laterally sited **medullary reticulospinal tract** originates largely on the same side, and its fibers end without crossing the midline. Reticulospinal fibers end by synapsing with interneurons, mainly in lamina VII.

The central nuclei of the reticular formation receive afferent fibers from the various **motor areas of the cerebral cortex,** and, by spinoreticular tracts, from the **spinal cord.** There are also fibers from the central nuclei of the **cerebellum.**

The reticulospinal tracts are thought to mediate the control of those movements that do not need conscious attention. Probably most movements would fall into this category. The corticospinal fibers provide a more direct route between the cerebral cortex and the motor neurons, perhaps providing the pathway normally used to make volitional movements. The effects of transection of the pyramid indicate, however, that the corticospinal fibers are indispensable only for skilled movements of the hands.

Vestibulospinal Tract

This tract (sometimes called the lateral vestibulospinal tract) originates from the **lateral vestibular nucleus** in the medulla. The fibers descend ipsilaterally and end on interneurons and motor neurons on the *same side* of the spinal cord. Stimulation of vestibulospinal neurons causes contraction of extensor muscles and relaxation of flexors—movements that oppose gravity and thereby contribute to the maintenance of an upright posture. The lateral vestibular nucleus receives its input from the **vestibular ganglion** and from the **vestibulocerebellum.** There are no cortico-vestibular connections.

If the brain stem is transected above the medulla, the uninhibited activity of vestibulospinal neurons causes **decerebrate rigidity.** In this condition the limbs are extended and the back is arched. The classical animal model of decerebrate rigidity is a cat with a transected midbrain. A comparable condition occurs in man if the neuraxis is severed rostral to the midbrain by the growth of a tumor.

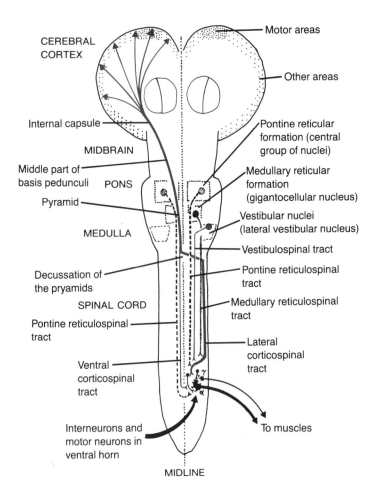

Figure 23-1 Descending tracts involved in the control of movement.

Rubrospinal Tract

Experimental work in cats and monkeys indicates that the red nucleus provides, in those species, an important link between the cerebral cortex and the motor neurons of the spinal cord. In man, however, the rubrospinal tract is tiny and extends no further caudally than segment C2 of the spinal cord. The largest contingent of descending fibers from the human red nucleus travels in the central tegmental tract and ends in the inferior olivary nucleus. This connection forms part of the circuitry of the cerebellum.

Upper and Lower Motor Neuron Paralysis

A **paralyzed** muscle does not do any useful work. A **paretic** muscle in weak; paresis is partial paralysis. Paralysis or paresis may be due to injury or disease affecting *either* the motor neurons that innervate muscles, *or* parts of the central nervous system directly involved in controlling the activities of the motor neurons. Muscular weakness from abnormality in the central nervous system is due to interruption of descending pathways. Paralysis and paresis must not be confused with other disorders of motor control (see Chap. 24) in which movements are abnormal but can be made with adequate strength.

The term **lower motor neuron,** used in clinical neurology, identifies the population of motor neurons that supplies any group of muscles. A **lower motor neuron lesion** is paralysis or weakness due either to destruction of the somata of the motor neurons or to loss of function of their axons. The axons may fail to conduct if they are transected or if their myelin sheaths are lost as a consequence of a peripheral neuropathy.

Muscles paralyzed by a lower motor neuron lesion are **flaccid,** and it is impossible to elicit contraction by stretching the tendons (**absent tendon jerk reflexes**). Electromyography reveals frequent random contractions of individual muscle fibers in denervated muscles. This condition is called **fibrillation;** it is detectable only by electrical recording.* After being denervated for a few weeks, a muscle becomes much smaller. This **denervation atrophy** is due partly to disuse and partly to loss of a specific myotrophic action of the motor neurons. The myotrophic effect is probably mediated by a protein synthesized by the neuron and released at the neuromuscular junction.

There is no such thing as an "upper motor neuron." However, it is convenient to recognize a clinical entity called an **upper motor neuron lesion.** This is a *syndrome* (see Chap. 21 for definition) in which paralysis or paresis is due to interruption of descending pathways. The causative lesion does not involve a specific population of neurons. Indeed the same abnormalities can result from destructive lesions in widely separate parts of the central nervous system.

Muscles paralyzed by an upper motor neuron lesion are **spastic,** owing to excessive activity of the stretch reflex. The **tendon jerks are exaggerated** for the same reason, and so is reflex withdrawal from a mildly painful stimulus applied to the skin. An important abnormal withdrawal reflex is the **Babinski response.** This consists of dorsiflexion of the big toe accompanied by flexion of the hip and knee joints when the sole of the foot is stroked with a hard object. This abnormal reflex is named after a French clinical neurologist, Joseph Babinski (1857–1932). The normal response to stroking the sole is plantar flexion of the big toe. The muscles paralyzed by an upper

---

* Visible twitching of small bundles of muscle fibers is **fasciculation.** This is common in partially denervated muscles, but it also frequently seen in normal people, so its diagnostic value is not great.

motor neuron lesion are not denervated, so there is no fibrillation and no denervation atrophy. The muscles do eventually become smaller from disuse, but this atrophy is slower and less severe than that of denervated muscles.

One cause of upper motor neuron paralysis is transection of the spinal cord, described at the beginning of this chapter. A much more common condition is infarction in a cerebral hemisphere, caused by arterial obstruction. Sudden paralysis due to obstruction of a cerebral artery is called a **stroke.** The area infarcted may be the cerebral cortex, in which case both the primary motor and premotor areas are usually involved, or it may be a small region within the internal capsule. These lesions produce *paralysis of the opposite side of the body.* If the spastic paralysis involves the upper and lower limbs together, it is called **hemiplegia.** Paralysis of both lower limbs from a spinal lesion is **paraplegia.** Paralysis of all four limbs from a lesion in the upper cervical spinal cord is called **tetraplegia.** (The suffix *-plegia* is the Greek for "a blow.")

The causes of the symptoms and signs of an upper motor neuron lesion are poorly understood because it is not known just which descending pathways must be interrupted to produce the condition. Certainly the syndrome does not result from selective transection of either the corticospinal or the vestibulospinal tract. This leaves the reticulospinal tracts as the only major descending pathways whose transection might be responsible. Lesions in the cerebral hemisphere might sever corticoreticular and corticospinal fibers. Lesions in the midbrain or medulla have to extend dorsally beyond the territory of the corticospinal fibers if they are to cause hemiplegia. It is probably reasonable to conclude that although most lesions causing upper motor neuron paralysis involve the corticospinal

tract, transected corticoreticular or reticulospinal fibers may account for most of the clinical features of the paralysis.

Some Outmoded Terminology That Still Causes Confusion

The clinical entity known as an "upper motor neuron lesion" is still sometimes called the "pyramidal tract syndrome," in the mistaken belief that the paralysis, spasticity, and Babinski's reflex are due only to transection of fibers of the pyramidal system. It has been known since the mid-1950s, however, that the consequences of cutting the pyramidal fibers are quite different from those of the common upper motor neuron lesion.

The expression "extrapyramidal system" was introduced many years ago for descending pathways other than the corticospinal and corticobulbar tracts. As an anatomical term, this would be unnecessary but reasonable. Clinical neurologists, however, recognize a variety of "extrapyramidal disorders" that are diseases in which there are unwanted involuntary movements. The lesions causing these diseases are in the basal ganglia, which do not send descending fibers to the spinal cord or cranial nerve nuclei. There is no reason to suspect that extrapyramidal disorders have anything to do with the reticulospinal or vestibulospinal tracts. The word "extrapyramidal" has done nothing but cause confusion, and it is not used in modern textbooks of neuroanatomy, neurophysiology or clinical neurology. Disorders characterized by involuntary movements are now called **dyskinesias** (from the Greek, "disordered or difficult movement"), a term that encompasses several different syndromes without presuming to identify their causes.

Chapter 24

Control of Movement
by the Cerebellum
and Basal Ganglia

The descending pathways described in Chapter 23 are used by the brain to issue commands to motor neurons. The formulation of the commands is carried out in several parts of the brain that do not give rise to descending tracts. The most important such parts are the **cerebellum** and the **basal ganglia.** Both recieve input from many sources; both direct most of their output through the thalamus to the motor areas of the cerebral cortex. Thus the motor cortex receives neural signals that have been processed by the cerebellum and basal ganglia, and it sends out, to the reticular formation and spinal cord, signals that determine which muscles will contract, how strongly, and for how long. Regions of the cerebral cortex other than the motor areas also influence the cerebellum and the basal ganglia, and there are association fibers that interconnect the various cortical areas. Thus the whole cortex contributes to the content of motor commands, and the motor areas channel the commands towards the neurons that supply the muscles Figure 24-1 summarizes these interconnections.

Cerebellum

The anatomy of the cerebellum is described in Chapter 9. Its major connections with other parts of the brain must now be considered.

Connections and Activities of the Cerebellum

All parts of the cerebellum receive climbing fiber afferents from the **inferior olivary complex of nuclei.** Fibers afferent to the olive come from several places, including the motor areas of the cerebral cortex, the red nucleus, and the spinal cord.

Axons from sites other than the inferior olivary complex end as mossy fibers in the cerebellum. The cerebellum has three divisions, the vestibulocerebellum, the spinocerebellum, and the pontocerebellum (see Chap. 9). These receive mossy fibers from different places and also have different efferent projections:

1. The **vestibulocerebellum** receives and transmits signals concerned with equilibration (see Chap. 17; also Fig. 24-2).
2. The **spinocerebellum** receives proprioceptive input and uses this to modify (1) the activity of the motor cortex, through the thalamus; and (2) the activity of the climbing fibers, through the red nucleus.
3. The **pontocerebellum** receives input from most of the neocortex through the pontine nuclei. Its output is directed, through the thalamus, to the first, second, and supplementary motor areas.

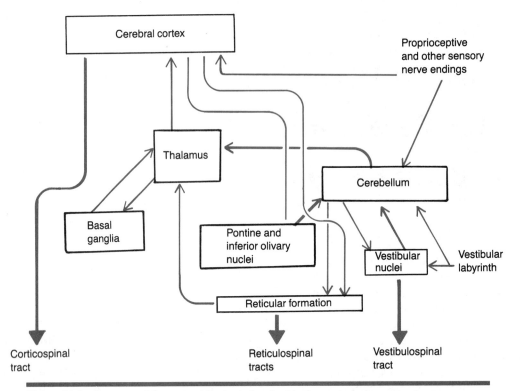

Figure 24-1   Summary of the parts of the brain involved in the control of movement.

The connections of the cerebellum are ordered such that each cerebellar hemisphere is connected with the same side of the body and with the contralateral cerebral hemisphere.

The major connections of the cerebellum are summarized in Figure 24-2. In learning about the control of movement, the student should also be familiar with the material in Chapters 9 and 23.

It is thought that the cerebellum stores instructions for patterns of movement that are frequently performed. The teaching of the patterns is done by the olivocerebellar neurons. The instruction to use a particular stored program enters the cerebellum through the mossy fibers. The different mossy fiber populations also enable the cerebellum to compare motor commands (ordering what should happen) with proprioceptive data (saying what did happen) so that refinements can be made to the signals issuing from the motor cortex.

Electrophysiological studies in monkeys indicate that when a movement is made the neurons in the dentate nucleus of the cerebellum are active *before* the neurons in the primary motor cortex. This observation does not mean that the cerebellum initiates movements; initiation is a function of many parts of the brain. It does show, however, that the primary motor cortex is not an area that thinks and directs movement, but rather a funnel through which other regions of the central nervous system send their contributions. The neurons in the supplementary motor area are active long before a movement is made. In man, merely thinking about a movement is accompanied by increased blood flow in the supplementary motor area.

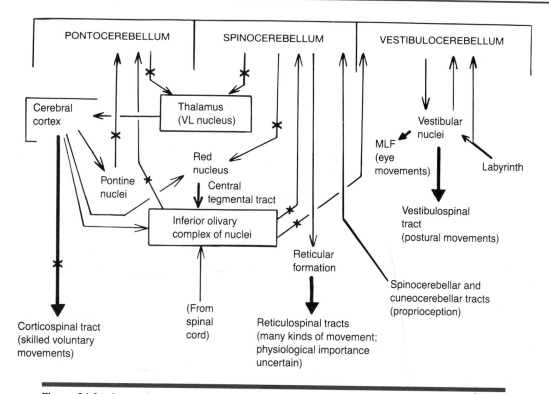

Figure 24-2 Connections of the three functional divisions (see Chap. 9) of the cerebellum, to show their influence on descending tracts. Crosses (×) indicate tracts that cross the midline. Each cerebellar hemisphere works in conjunction with the same side of the body and with the contralateral cerebral hemisphere. It is the posterior division of the VL thalamic nucleus that receives input from the cerebellar nuclei, and its projection is principally to the primary motor area.

Cerebellar Disorders

When the cerebellum is not working properly, there is inadequate control of the timing and range of movement, with resulting clumsiness. The condition is known as **ataxia,** a word which in Greek means "loss of order." Ataxia can also be due to loss of proprioceptive sensation, but then other sensory deficits are apparent too. The manifestations of cerebellar ataxia vary with the part of the cerebellum that is abnormal. The two typical syndromes are that due to lesions in and near the midline, and that due to lesions in the lateral parts of the hemisphere.

Damage in the midline of the cerebellum of a child is usually due to a medulloblastoma,

a malignant tumor arising from neuroglial cells in that region. In adults, chronic alcoholism can result in degeneration of the median and medial parts of the cerebellum. Both the vestibulocerebellum and the spinocerebellum are involved in these conditions, so the abnormalities are of equilibration and gait. The failure of coordination of contractions of muscles affects those movements most dependent on vestibular sensation and proprioceptive feedback. Consequently the patient walks unsteadily, with the feet widely spaced. It is difficult to turn or to stop quickly. The term "truncal ataxia" is sometimes applied to this disorder. The movements of the limbs for purposes other than locomotion are well coordinated.

Damage to the lateral part of the cerebellar hemisphere may be due to a tumor or to occlusion of an artery. The ataxia is seen in movements of *the same side of the body,* as predicted from the connections of the pontocerebellum. Skilled movements cannot be carried out. The amount of movement is inappropriate, so the hand overshoots on the first attempt to touch anything, especially at arm's length. This is called "past-pointing." A coarse tremor is present, often only when movements are being made; it is called "intention tremor." (This tremor is often found in multiple sclerosis. Demyelination of dentatothalamic fibers in the brain stem may be the cause of intention tremor rather than disease in the cerebellum itself.) There are several other tests of the function of the pontocerebellum. The best known is to ask the patient to make rapidly alternating rotations of the wrists. If only slow, jerky movements can be made, there is "dysdiadochokinesis." This rather pretentious word is made up from Greek components that mean "difficulty with successive movement."

Several rare disorders, including some inherited degenerative diseases of the brain, cause bilateral mixed abnormalities of the different functional parts of the cerebellum.

The Basal Ganglia

The term "basal ganglia" refers to the **corpus striatum,** together with the **subthalamic nucleus** and the **substantia nigra.** Diseases that disrupt these interconnected structures cause derangements of movement known as **dyskinesias.** Unfortunately, there is no obvious relationship between the neuroanatomy and the effects of lesions. Neither is it possible to attribute simple normal functions to the basal ganglia; they may well be involved in other cerebral activities in addition to the control of movement.

Connections and Activities of the Basal Ganglia

The most conspicuous connections of the basal ganglia are summarized in Figure 24-3. Many others are known. Perhaps the most important general trend in the connections is convergence from many parts of the brain to the motor areas of the cerebral cortex, in a loop that passes through the corpus striatum. The other nuclei have two-way connections with parts of the corpus striatum. Some of the neurotransmitters used in the basal ganglia are known, and this knowledge has led to useful new drugs for the treatment of one disease of the system.

Electrical recordings indicate that the neostriatum, like the pontocerebellum, is active a few milliseconds *before* a movement is made. At this time, the neostriatal neurons become active and inhibit the paleostriatal (pallidal) neurons. The latter cells fire most frequently when no movement is being made. The pallidal neurons, being GABAergic, inhibit the thalamic neurons upon which their axons terminate. Inhibition of the GABAergic pallidum by the GABAergic principal cells of the neostriatum thus results in more impulses being sent from the thalamus to the motor cortex. The thalamocortical neurons are excitatory. The principal cells of the motor cortical areas are thus stimulated by input from the pontocerebellum and basal ganglia, and presumably also from other areas of the cerebral cortex. Modifications affecting the precision of movements in progress occur through edited proprioceptive signals from the spinocerebellum.

The rate of firing of nigrostriatal dopaminergic neurons is steady and does not vary with movement. The action of the dopamine is to inhibit both the cholinergic (excitatory) interneurons and the GABAergic principal cells of the neostriatum. Loss of dopaminergic nigral neurons causes Parkinson's disease (see below). The way in which normality of

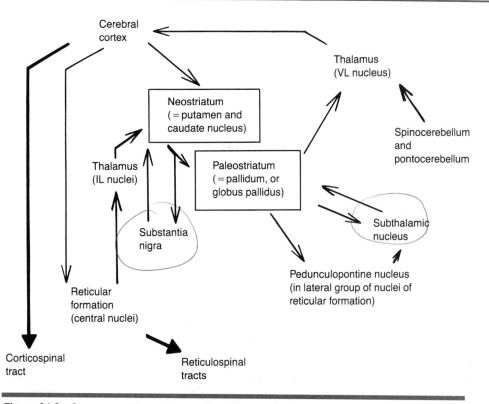

Figure 24-3 Some connections of the corpus striatum and other components of the basal ganglia. The neostriatum receives input from the whole neocortex. The pallidum projects to the anterior division of the VL, and the projection from this thalamic nucleus is principally to the premotor area.

movements is ensured by constant discharge from the substantia nigra is not known. Dopamine may act as a neuromodulator (see Chap. 3), affecting the responses of the neostriatal neurons to classical neurotransmitters used by their other sources of afferent fibers.

Dyskinesias

The Greek components of dyskinesia mean "difficult movement." These disorders are associated with unwanted extra muscular contractions.

Parkinson's disease* is the most common dyskinesia. It is due to degeneration of do-

---

* James Parkinson (1775–1824), an Englishman, was a paleontologist as well as a physician and surgeon.

paminergic neurons of the substantia nigra. The most serious feature of the condition is *akinesia* or "poverty of movement." There is difficulty in initiating movement (and in stopping), and a lack of associated movements such as swinging the arms when walking or holding the head erect when sitting. Loss of the involuntary movements of the face causes a masklike expression, and smiling or frowning can be done only as a deliberate act. The other abnormalities are muscular *rigidity,* typically with intermittent ("cogwheel") resistance to passive movements of joints, and a slow *tremor* of the fingers, forearms, jaw, and head. The tremor is present at rest and disappears when a movement is being made. In this respect it is the converse of a cerebellar tremor.

All three major abnormalities in Parkinson's disease are alleviated by treatment with L-dopa (*levodopa*), the metabolic precursor of dopamine. The drug is converted into dopamine, probably by surviving nigral dopaminergic neurons, and inhibits the abnormal overactivity of the neostriatum. Anticholinergic drugs such as *benzhexol* and *ethopropazine* inhibit the actions of cholinergic interneurons upon the principal cells of the neostriatum. Anticholinergic drugs reduce the tremor and rigidity, but not the akinesia. Tremor and rigidity can also be relieved by surgical placement of destructive lesions in the pallidum or the VL nucleus of the thalamus. Surgery is now rarely needed, however, because L-dopa is usually just as effective and has the added advantage of relieving the akinesia. Unfortunately, drugs or operations have no effect on the progress of the disease, the cause of which is unknown. Eventually the akinesia becomes severely disabling, and other changes in the brain lead, in many patients, to loss of mental capabilities. Failure of the mind due to disease of the brain is called **dementia.** Some possible anatomical correlates of dementia are discussed in Chapter 25.

Loss of neurons in the caudate nucleus and putamen (together constituting the striatum or neostriatum) causes **chorea.** In this dyskinesia, there are spontaneous, irregular contractions of groups of muscles, especially in the face and upper limbs. The movements are absent in sleep. **Sydenham's chorea,**[†] also called St. Vitus's dance, is an unusual response to a certain strain of *Streptococcus*. **Huntington's chorea**[§] is an inherited degenerative disease of the neostriatum. Symptoms appear in middle age, and the chorea is associated with progressive dementia.

Athetosis is associated with degeneration of both the neo-‌ and the paleostriatum. Large writhing movements of the limbs occur, complicating and frustrating the intended movements. The commonest cause is injury to the brain at birth as a result of physical distortion, oxygen deficiency, or other metabolic disturbance. Athetoid movements are a common feature of **cerebral palsy.** Afflicted children often respond well to intensive training ("conductive education"), because their mental abilities are not impaired by the abnormality in the corpus striatum. Other types of cerebral palsy consist of upper motor neuron lesions (see Chapter 24), with spastic paralysis or paresis of two or four limbs. There may be mental retardation, too, if large areas of cortex have degenerated.

Hemiballismus consists of large, purposeless movements of the upper and lower limbs, contralateral to a destructive lesion in the subthalamic nucleus. The usual cause is an arterial occlusion. The patient may die, but recovery is more usual. Hemiballismus can be relieved by surgical transection of the corticospinal fibers in the basis pedunculi. As explained in Chapter 23, this does not cause hemiplegia.

Several other dyskinesias are known. Some are unwanted effects of antipsychotic drugs, notably certain phenothiazines and butyrophenones. These conditions are sometimes called "extrapyramidal syndromes," but this confusing and meaningless term should not be used (see Chap. 23).

The student may also be interested to know that "chorea" is from the Greek for "dance," and that "athetosis" in Greek would mean "without position." "Hemiballismus," also of Greek origin, indicates the jumping or throwing (ballism) of half (hemi-) the body.

[†] Thomas Sydenham (1624–1689), also English, was one of the first physicians to apply logical principles to diagnosis and therapy.

[§] George S. Huntington (1850–1916) was a general medical practitioner in the United States.

Chapter 25

The Limbic System

The term **limbic system** is used in various ways by different authors. Here it is used in its widest possible sense, to include the hippocampal formation, the cortex of the limbic lobe (see below), and all the associated tracts and subcortical regions.

Gray Matter of the Limbic System

The Limbic Cortex

The name "limbic" was coined by Pierre Broca (see Chap. 22) from the Latin *limbus,* meaning a hem or border. Broca's "limbic lobe" is a ring of cortex around the corpus callosum and cerebral penduncle. Reference to Figure 11-1 in Chapter 11 will show that the limbic lobe consists of the **cingulate** and **parahippocampal gyri,** which are connected behind the corpus callosum and across the septal area and the limen insulae. The cortex of the parahippocampal gyrus extends medially and dorsally to become rolled inside the temporal lobe as the **hippocampus.** The anatomy is best appreciated by following the cortical surface on a coronal (transverse) section. The term **hippocampal formation** includes the hippocampus itself, together with the closely associated **dentate gyrus** and the white matter of the **alveus, fimbria,** and **fornix** (Fig. 25-1).

The name "hippocampus" is from a fanciful resemblance to a sea horse (Greek). The dentate gyrus is so named because it looks rather like a row of teeth between the fimbria and the parahippocampal gyrus. The thin layer of white matter on the surface of the hippocampus is called the *alveus,* although its relationship to a trough (Latin) is obscure. *Fimbria* is Latin for "fringe" and is descriptive of the ridge formed by the gathering together of the axons from the alveus. The fimbria continues into the **fornix** (from the Latin for "arch"). The fornices of the two sides meet with exchange of some axons above the roof of the third ventricle. On each side the fornices then diverge, eventually to enter the septal area and the hypothalamus. The rostral (anterior) end of the parahippocampal gyrus is the **entorhinal area,** so named because it is medial to the rhinal sulcus. Medial to the entorhinal area is the uncus (see Chap. 14). The entorhinal area serves as association cortex for olfaction and is thus a site of overlap between the limbic and olfactory systems. ("Rhinal" is an adjective derived from the Greek for "nose.")

The cortex of the "limbic lobe" is connected by association fibers with the cortex of the **temporal pole** (the anterior or rostral end of the temporal lobe) and with the cortex of the **orbital surface of the frontal lobe.** The cingulate gyrus is connected with the **anterior group of thalamic nuclei,** and the orbitofrontal cortex with the **mediodorsal nucleus** of the thalamus. (For more about thalamic nuclei, see Chap. 10.)

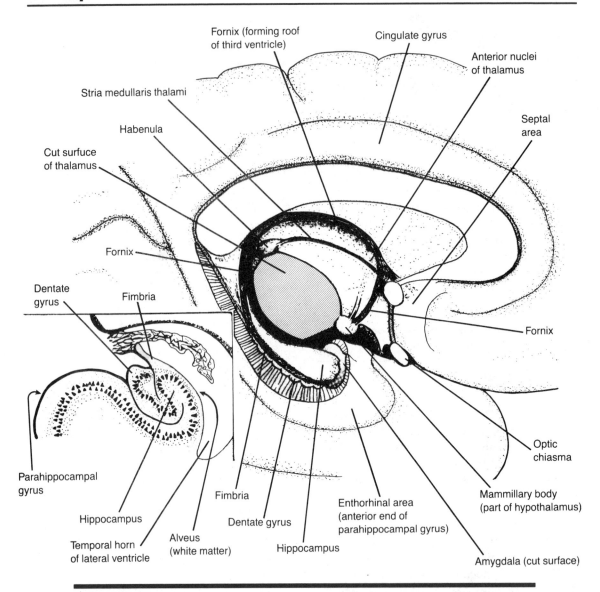

Figure 25-1   The medial surface of the left cerebral hemisphere, which has been removed by cutting through the thalamus. Part of the temporal lobe has been removed to open the temporal horn of the lateral ventricle and expose the hippocampus and amygdala. The parts of the limbic system are labeled. Dissection in the wall of the third ventricle shows the termination of the fornix and part of the trajectory of the mammillothalamic tract. The inset in the lower left corner is a simplified drawing of a transverse (coronal) section through the temporal lobe. It shows the position of the hippocampal formation in relation to the lateral ventricle and the parahippocampal gyrus. The choroid plexus is invaginated into the ventricle, alongside the fimbria and fornix (compare with Fig. 30-1).

Other Limbic Structures

Two thalamic nuclei have already been mentioned. Other parts of the diencephalon included in the limbic system are the **mammillary bodies,** most of the other nuclei of the **hypothalamus,** and the **habenular nuclei** of the epithalamus.

Subcortical structures in the forebrain are also involved in the limbic circuitry. The **septal area** is inferior (ventral) to the recurved rostral end of the corpus callosum. The septal area is next to the preoptic area, which is part of the forebrain, though its connections are similar to those of the nearby anterior hypothalamus. The *nucleus accumbens septi,* despite its name, is not part of the septal area. It is the most ventral part of the putamen, and its connections are those of the neostriatum (Chaps. 11, and 24).

Another major telencephalic limbic structure is the **amygdala** (Latin for an almond), also known as the amygdaloid body. This is rostral and medial to the tip of the temporal horn of the lateral ventricle. On the medial surface of the temporal lobe, the amygdala blends into the cortex of the uncus. Several nuclei are present in the amygdala, but they are not described in this book. Let it suffice to say that the *corticomedial nuclei* receive input from the olfactory tract, whereas the *basolateral* and *central* groups of nuclei receive afferent fibers from the neocortex of the temporal lobe and belong to the limbic system.

Ascending fibers reach the telencephalic limbic structures from the **ventral tegmental area** of the midbrain, the **locus ceruleus** (blue place) in the pons, and the **raphe nuclei** of the brain stem. The rostral parts of the limbic system send fibers caudally to the **reticular formation,** the **cranial nerve nuclei** (mainly X), and the **spinal cord.** In addition, there are extensive corticocortical connections in the cerebral hemispheres.

Connections of the Limbic System

To simplify the circuitry, three sets of connections will be described: those intrinsic to the telencephalic and diencephalic parts of the limbic system, and the pathways leading into and out of the intrinsic circuitry.

Connections Confined to the Telencephalon and Diencephalon

The American comparative neuroanatomist James W. Papez (1883–1958) suggested in 1937 that the hippocampus, the hypothalamus, the anterior thalamic nuclei, and their interconnections might be involved in the subjective feeling of emotions and in the expression of emotions through the somatic motor and autonomic nervous systems.

The word "emotion" is extremely difficult to define, especially for animals that cannot talk. In neuroscience emotions are usually considered to be activities in the brain that result in actions necessary for survival. For example, fear is an experience that might result from any of a variety of sensory stimuli. The effects of fear may include such activities as running away, keeping still, or fighting. These activities are associated with responses of the autonomic and endocrine systems, such as increased cardiac output, vasodilatation in muscles, increased concentration of glucose in the blood, and the functionally related (though not autonomically mediated) provision of more oxygen by acceleration of respiratory movements. Other effects of fear, with less obvious values for survival, may include evacuation of the urinary bladder and colon, sweating, and pupillary dilatation. Other incentives that drive emotional responses include the activities of the central nervous system in hunger, thirst, pain, adverse environmental temperature, and the proximity of a potential mate or rival. The reason for the adaptive behavior in response to any of these circumstances is called "motivation." Motivation depends not only upon the necessity for action but also on learned experience.

The connections implicated by Papez in emotional feeling and expression are customarily called **"Papez' circuit"** (Fig. 25-2). Of course, a simple circular array of neurons could be used only in conjunction with suitable pathways leading in and out of the circuit. These are described later in this chapter.

Many connections of the **amygdala** are confined to the telencephalon and the diencephalon, though there is probably not a closed loop equivalent to Papez' circuit. The connections shown in Figure 25-3 are the most conspicuous. The input and output of the system shown will be described presently. The *stria terminalis* is a slender tract that follows the curve of the lateral ventricle, between the caudate nucleus and thalamus. The *diagonal band* lies deep to the anterior perforated substance. The *ventral amygdalofugal pathway* is ventral (inferior) to the lentiform nucleus, following the most direct route from the tem-

poral lobe to the thalamus, posterior (caudal) to the diagonal band.

Input to the Limbic System

Subcortical *association fibers* interconnect all areas of the cerebral cortex, including that of the temporal pole, which is the largest source of fibers afferent to the entorhinal area (of the parahippocampal gyrus) and the amygdala. Thus the hippocampus and the other components of the circuits shown in Figures 25-1 and 25-2 are probably influenced by the **whole cerebral cortex,** with a funnelling of the input through the temporal pole.

Ascending fibers in the *fornix,* the *stria terminalis,* and the *medial forebrain bundle* come from the **ventral tegmental area** (the "mesolimbic dopaminergic system"), the **locus ceruleus** (noradrenergic neurons), the **raphe nuclei** (serotonergic neurons), the **parabrachial nucleus** (see Chap. 21), and the **solitary nucleus** (Chap. 20, 27). These afferent fibers end in the hippocampal formation, amygdala, hypothalamus, septal area, and prefrontal cor-

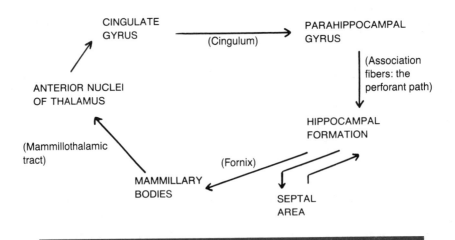

Figure 25-2 The circuit of Papez. (The lateral dorsal nucleus and some other thalamic nuclei [see Chap. 10] have connections similar to those of the anterior nuclear group.)

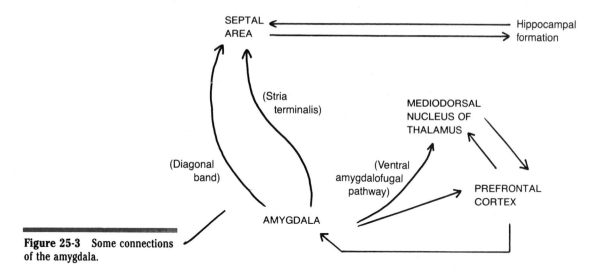

Figure 25-3 Some connections of the amygdala.

tex. The fornix also carries axons to the hippocampal formation from the **septal area** (cholinergic), the **hypothalamus,** various **thalamic nuclei** (see Chap. 10), and the **substantia innominata** (see later in this chapter).

Disordered activity of neurons with axons ascending to the limbic system is postulated in some mental diseases, notably **schizophrenia.** The principal supporting evidence is that certain drugs valuable in the treatment of schizophrenic patients are blockers of dopamine receptors. A similar theory 'attributes **depression** to insufficient activity of ascending noradrenergic and serotonergic fibers. Antidepressive drugs either mimic or potentiate the actions of noradrenaline and serotonin.

Output of the Limbic System

The parts of the limbic system in the forebrain contain neurons with axons that end in the neocortex, and neurons with axons that project caudally.

The output to the **neocortex** is through association fibers, which connect the parahippocampal gyrus, the cingulate gyrus, and the

prefrontal cortex with all other parts of the cerebral cortex.

The descending output of the limbic system is channelled through pathways that originate in the septal area and the hypothalamus:

1. The **stria medullaris thalami** (see Chap. 10) originates in the septal area. The axons terminate in the **habenular nuclei** of the epithalamus. The axons of the habenular neurons form, on each side, the **fasciculus retroflexus** (from the Latin, meaning "a bundle bent back"). The fasciculi retroflexi end in the **interpeduncular nucleus** in the midline of the ventral part of the tegmentum of the midbrain. The interpeduncular nucleus projects to more caudal parts of the reticular formation.

2. The **mammillotegmental tract** consists of caudally directed branches of mammillothalamic fibers. The tract goes to dorsal parts of the tegmentum of the midbrain.

3. The **medial forebrain bundle** contains fibers of many different lengths running rostrally and caudally. The bundle includes the axons of septal neurons that pass into the hypothalamus and into the tegmen-

tum of the midbrain. Hypothalamotegmental fibers are also present. The medial forebrain bundle passes through and has its connections with the lateral parts of the hypothalamus.

4. The **dorsal longitudinal fasciculus** arises from the amygdala and from the medial parts of the hypothalamus. Its fibers descend ventral to the cerebral aqueduct and then near the midline in the floor of the fourth ventricle. Some continue further caudally as a **hypothalamospinal tract.** The fibers of this system terminate around the cells of origin of preganglionic autonomic fibers, especially in the dorsal nucleus of the vagus and the spinal gray matter in segments T1-L3, and S2-S4.

5. Inasmuch as it originates in the hypothalamus, the **hypothalamo-hypophysial tract** must be considered an efferent pathway of the limbic system, permitting a pervasive influence of many parts of the forebrain upon the endocrine system.

Disorders of the Limbic System

The postulated functions of the human limbic system are deduced from the effects of destructive lesions. Such *lesions must be bilateral in order to cause symptoms.*

Korsakoff's psychosis, * seen in alcoholics and perhaps due to associated deficiency of thiamine (vitamin B_1), has been attributed to bilateral lesions in the mammillary bodies and in the mediodorsal thalamic nuclei. The principal clinical feature is inability to recall newly acquired memories. Typically the patient makes up fictitious answers to questions

* Sergei Sergeivich Korsakoff (1854–1900) was a Russian psychiatrist.

when the answers require recently remembered information. The defect of memory is not the only component of the syndrome. Lesions that destroy both hippocampal formations are rare, but do cause failure of the remembering mechanism. These clinical findings agree with the results of animal experiments in which lesions interrupt Papez' circuit bilaterally.

Failure to remember recent experiences occurs in various diseases that cause dementia, including the commonest cause of senility, **Alzheimer's disease.** * In this condition there are degenerative changes in the hippocampi and in a group of neurons at the base of the forebrain, in an area bounded by the hypothalamus medially, the corpus striatum dorsally, and the amygdala laterally. This area is the **substantia innominata,** and the neurons that degenerate in Alzheimer's disease are large ones constituting the **basal nucleus** of Meynert.[†] In normal monkeys, these large neurons are cholinergic and have neurons that branch profusely and end in all areas of the cerebral cortex. Chemical and immunocytochemical evidence points to the existence of equivalent connections in man, but it is not known if loss of cholinergic innervation of the cortex is responsible for any of the mental changes in Alzheimer's disease. In advanced cases there is considerable degeneration of the cortex itself, with conspicuous shrinkage of the gyri. It has been postulated that the cortical atrophy is due to transneuronal degeneration following loss of the cholinergic afferent fibers from the basal nucleus.

Some very rare lesions provide support for the notion that accumulation of memory oc-

* Alois Alzheimer (1864–1915) was a German pioneer of neuropathology.
† T.H. Meynert (1833–1902) was an Austrian clinical neurologist, best known for his contributions to neuroanatomy.

curs in the temporal lobe. Thus there is failure to remember newly seen events or places if the occipitotemporal association fibers are bilaterally severed. A corresponding inability to remember recent spoken words can follow bilateral lesions that disconnect the entorhinal area from the auditory association cortex.

The **amygdala** has been electrically stimulated in patients undergoing surgery under local anesthesia. They describe feelings of fear and, occasionally, of anger. Stimulation in cats or monkeys causes furious defensive behavior, with aggressive gestures and noises and activity of all parts of the sympathetic nervous system (see Chap. 27). Similar activity follows stimulation of the lateral hypothalamus in animals. Bilateral destruction of the amygdala makes cats and monkeys docile, and has occasionally been carried out successfully as treatment for a rare human disorder in which there are episodes of irrational and uncontrollable rage. (Attacks of rage can also be due to hypothyroidism, an easily treated endocrine deficiency.)

The hippocampus and the amygdala are both in the temporal lobe, a part of the brain in which **epileptic attacks** often originate. The aura of such an attack (see Chap. 22) often involves peculiar feelings of memory or mood, together with unpleasant visceral sensations and manifestations of autonomic activity.

The changes following lesions that destroy the **orbitofrontal cortex,** or the fibers connecting it with the thalamus, are described in Chapter 22.

Functions of the Limbic System

Experimental and clinical observations support the view that the structures in the circuit of Papez are essential for the *remembering of recently acquired information.* In no disease is there a selective loss of the ability to recall facts that have been remembered for a long time. Old memories are therefore probably stored diffusely in the brain. The inferior surface of the temporal lobe, however, is concerned with storage or recall of old visual memories (see Chaps. 18 and 22).

The ascending input to the limbic system may govern, in a general way, the neural processes underlying certain *mental states:* rational thought and the degree of happiness or depression.

Through its descending pathways, the limbic system may act as a mediator between conscious thought (attributed vaguely to the neocortex) and the *involuntary activities* of the autonomic nervous system and endocrine glands, and immediate behavioral responses to danger.

With better understanding of the physiology of the nervous system, it may be necessary to abandon the idea of a "system" centered around the anatomical "limbic lobe." In the present state of knowledge, however, it is impossible to identify distinct units of neuronal circuitry for the functions of memory, emotion, and activity concerned with survival.

Chapter 26

The Hypothalamus

and its Activities

A simple description of the anatomy of the hypothalamus and hypophysis is given in Chapter 10, and several neural pathways connecting with this part of the brain are mentioned in connection with the closely associated limbic system in Chapter 25. This chapter is also concerned with connections of the hypothalamus, but more especially with its functions.

Input to the Hypothalamus

There are neurons in the hypothalamus that respond directly to changes in temperature of the blood, osmolarity of the plasma, and concentrations of circulating substances, notably hormones. Thus the hypothalamus is a sensory organ. There are also afferent nerve fibers from many parts of the central nervous system.

Summary of Neural Afferents

Nerve fibers enter the hypothalamus in the following tracts:

1. The **fornix,** carrying axons of hippocampal neurons, which end in the mammillary bodies and elsewhere.
2. The **medial forebrain bundle** brings fibers from the septal area and from the brain stem. The ascending afferents include fibers from the ventral tegmental area of the midbrain, the locus ceruleus, and the central nuclei of the reticular formation.
3. The **stria terminalis** and the **ventral amygdalofugal pathway** carry axons from the amygdala. Some of these fibers end in the hypothalamus.

The pathways conveying visceral sensory information to the hypothalamus are often presumed to be polysynaptic. In animals, however, some neurons in the solitary nucleus (see Chap. 20) are known to project directly to the hypothalamus and to the amygdala.

Output of the Hypothalamus

One major group of efferent hypothalamic connections is that consisting of neurosecretory axons that end on blood vessels of the hypophysis. Hypothalamic neurons also send axons to other parts of the central nervous system.

Summary of the Neural Efferents

The following tracts contain axons of neurons whose somata are in the hypothalamus.

1. The **hypothalamohypophysial fibers** will be discussed later in this chapter.
2. The **medial forebrain bundle,** which passes through the lateral part of the hypothalamus, includes fibers that go rostrally to the septal area and caudally to the tegmentum of the midbrain.
3. The **mammillothalamic tract,** part of the limbic system, projects to the anterior nuclear group of the thalamus.
4. The **mammillotegmental tract** is formed by branches of the axons that form the mammillothalamic tract. The caudally directed branches end in the dorsal part of the tegmentum of the midbrain.
5. The **dorsal longitudinal fasciculus** contains the axons of neurons in the medial part of the hypothalamus. The tract goes to groups of preganglionic autonomic neurons, notably the dorsal nucleus of the vagus, the lateral horn of spinal gray matter in segments T1 to L2 and the sacral autonomic nucleus in segments S2 to S4 of the spinal cord.

Nonendocrine Hypothalamic Functions

Thermoregulation

The temperature-sensitive neurons are in the anterior hypothalamic area, which by indirect routes also receives edited neural information from temperature-sensitive nerve endings in the skin. The hypothalamic neurons direct the activities of the autonomic nervous system. Regulatory neurons that counteract increased temperature reside predominantly in the anterior part of the hypothalamus, whereas the posterior area contains neurons whose activities prevent the temperature from falling. The efferent pathway from the anterior thermoregulatory neurons passes through the posterior hypothalamic area. Consequently a destructive lesion in the anterior part of the hypothalamus causes an uncontrolled rise in the temperature of the body, but a lesion in the posterior hypothalamic area impairs all temperature regulation.

The regulation of temperature by the hypothalamus is mediated mainly by controlling the loss of heat. In man, therefore, the most important action is directed upon the preganglionic neurons of the sympathetic division of the autonomic system (see Chap. 27). Postganglionic sympathetic neurons supply the blood vessels and eccrine sweat glands of the skin. Hypothalamic influences on motor neurons increase heat production by shivering when the surrounding environment is cold. In furry animals the sympathetically innervated piloarrector muscles provide a thicker insulating layer of air in the coat. In people the equivalent muscles produce goose pimples, which provide no obvious functional benefit.

Osmoregulation

The osmotic pressure of the plasma of the blood is determined mainly by the concentrations of dissolved sodium and chloride ions. The concentrations of these and other solutes must be kept within narrow limits of tolerance. The stabilization of the composition of the plasma is done largely by the kidneys. The hypothalamus contributes importantly, however, by controlling (a) the secretion of vasopressin, a hormone acting on the kidneys, and (b) drinking behavior.

Neurons that respond to changes in the osmotic pressure of the plasma are present in the lateral part of the hypothalamus and in the supraoptic nucleus. Increased osmotic pressure stimulates secretion of vasopressin, as described later in this chapter. Receptors in the walls of large veins respond to changes in the volume of blood returning to the heart.

Decreased volume signals to the hypothalamus the need for increased drinking, which is subjectively experienced as thirst. The hypothalamus also responds to circulating levels of angiotensin. This peptide is produced from a protein precursor in the plasma when the juxtaglomerular cells of the kidney secrete renin, a proteolytic enzyme. Renin is secreted if the supply of blood or oxygen to the kidney is reduced. Angiotensin has several actions, including:

1. Contraction of arterioles, thus raising arterial blood pressure
2. Stimulation of the adrenal cortex to secrete aldosterone, a hormone that makes the kidney retain sodium
3. Effects in the brain that result in thirst and drinking. Neurons responsive to angiotensin occur in the hypothalamus and also in the **subfornical organ** and the **area postrema** (Chap. 30), which send axons to the hypothalamus through the fornix

The lateral hypothalamic area and the nearby zona incerta (part of the subthalamus) are essential for control of water intake: Electrical stimulation in animals leads to excessive drinking, whereas bilateral destructive lesions cause dehydration.

Hunger and Satiety

Knowledge of hypothalamic involvement in feeding is derived largely from experiments in animals. Stimulation of the lateral hypothalamus causes eating, perhaps by making the animal feel hungry. Stimulation medially, in the anterior hypothalamic area, inhibits eating, perhaps by giving the animal a sense of being adequately fed (satiety). Destructive lesions have the opposite effect, but must be bilateral to cause abnormal behavior. Thus destruction of the ventral part of the anterior hypothalamic areas of both sides is followed by excessive eating that leads to obesity. Bilateral lesions laterally in the hypothalamus can result in failure to eat.

The feeling of hunger is partly a conscious awareness of emptiness of the stomach, but a more important factor may be a low concentration of glucose in the blood. There are hypothalamic neurons that respond to circulating levels of glucose and of cholecystokinin, a peptide hormone secreted by the intestine after feeding.

Although the ventral part of the anterior hypothalamic area is a satiety center in experimental animals, electrical stimulation of the equivalent region in man causes an ill-defined but decidedly unpleasant experience. Feelings of pleasure are induced by stimulation of the preoptic or septal area. Rats also seem to derive enjoyment from stimulation of these regions or of certain lateral hypothalamic sites. The animals quickly learn to press a bar that switches on the stimulator and will do this in preference to eating or drinking. The electrical stimuli in such experiments affect not only nuclei but axons of the medial forebrain bundle, which carry many limbic and hypothalamic connections. Anatomical knowledge of neuronal circuitry concerned with nasty and pleasing feelings is therefore still scanty.

Endocrine Functions of the Hypothalamus

The pituitary gland is controlled by **neurosecretory** cells of the hypothalamus. The axons of these neurons end in contact with capillary blood vessels in the **median eminence** and **posterior lobe** (see Chap. 10 for terminology). There the neurosecretory products are stored in axonal varicosities and boutons and released into the blood. Release is effected by the conduction of impulses along the axons.

The cells of the **anterior lobe** respond to **re-**

leasing hormones (also called "releasing factors") discharged into the capillaries of the median eminence. These vessels join up to form the **hypophysial portal system** of veins (Fig. 26-1). The portal veins empty into the capillary network of the anterior lobe of the gland. In this way neurosecretory products are carried in high concentrations from the median eminence to the cells that secrete the anterior pituitary hormones. The anterior and posterior lobes of the pituitary gland are drained by veins that lead into the cavernous sinus (see Chaps. 29, 30) and thence into the general circulation.

Posterior Lobe Hormones

Two hormones, **vasopressin** (also called **antidiuretic hormone, ADH**) and **oxytocin,** are synthesized in separate cells in the **supraoptic and** **paraventricular nuclei** of the hypothalamus. Following anterograde transport in the unmyelinated axons of the **hypothalamo-hypophysial tract,** the hormones are stored in and released from axonal varicosities and boutons in the posterior lobe.

Vasopressin promotes the passive absorption of water from the distal convoluted tubules and collecting tubules of the kidney, thereby reducing the volume of urine excreted. This antidiuretic action accounts for the hormone's alternative name. Unphysiologically large doses of ADH increase the arterial blood pressure (vasopressor action), and it is possible that the hormones may play a minor role in the normal control of peripheral blood vessels.

A hypothalamic lesion that transects the axons leading towards the pituitary stalk prevents the secretion of ADH, and large volumes of dilute urine are passed. This disease is

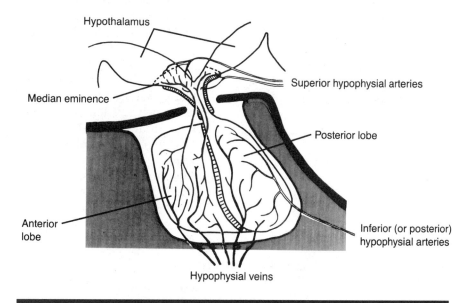

Figure 26-1 Vasculature of the pituitary gland. The **hypophysial portal veins,** which carry blood from the median eminence to the anterior lobe, are colored. The **hypophysial arteries** are branches of the internal carotids. The **hypophysial veins** drain into the cavernous sinuses (described in Chaps. 28 and 29). For anatomy and nomenclature of the hypothalamo-hypophysial system, see Fig. 10-4.

called **diabetes insipidus** because the urine is tasteless. A much more common condition is diabetes mellitus, in which a high concentration of glucose in the blood causes the passing of copious sugary urine. Diabetes mellitus is typically due to failure of the pancreatic islets to secrete insulin, the hormone that lowers the circulating levels of glucose.

Oxytocin receives its name from its action in causing contraction of the uterus. Another action of the same hormone is upon the myo-epithelial cells of the mammary gland. These contractile cells surround groups of milk-secreting cells, and their contraction squeezes milk into the ducts, an event known as **milk ejection** or letdown. Stimulation of the skin of the nipple by the infant's mouth initiates a spinohypothalamic reflex that causes secretion of oxytocin.

In the first few days after delivery, the secretion of oxytocin evoked by suckling also causes strong contractions of the uterus, thereby contributing to the shrinkage ("involution") of this organ. Prompt involution of the uterus prevents bleeding from the former site of attachment of the placenta.

Oxytocin is often used in obstetric practice to stimulate uterine contractions during labor. It is not known if secretion of oxytocin contributes normally to the emptying of the pregnant uterus. Labor is a complicated process involving many substances that act upon the uterine musculature.

Anterior Lobe Hormones

The pars distalis (see Chap. 10) secretes six hormones with well-established functions. Various names, all more or less self-explanatory, are given to these substances, which are all proteins.

1. **Corticotrophin** (adrenocorticotrophic hormone, **ACTH**) stimulates cells in the adrenal cortex that produce the glucocorticoids, the steroid hormones that affect carbohydrate metabolism. **Cortisol** (hydrocortisone) is the principal human glucocorticoid.

2. **Thyrotrophin** (thyrotrophic hormone, **TSH**) stimulates synthesis and secretion of thyroxine and triiodothyronine by the thyroid gland.

3. **Growth hormone** (somatotrophin, **STH**) acts mainly upon the liver, stimulating the secretion of **somatomedins.** The somatomedins are peptides that have numerous actions upon other cells. The most conspicuous effects of STH result in addition of bulk to bones and other organs.

4. **Follicle stimulating hormone (FSH)** stimulates the growth of the ovarian follicle and secretion of **estrogens.** In the male, FSH induces the Sertoli* cells of the testis to synthesize a protein that binds androgens. The principal androgen is **testosterone.**

5. **Luteinizing hormone (LH)** induces ovulation and the development of a corpus luteum in the ovary. The corpus luteum is stimulated by LH to secrete **progesterone.** In the male, LH is called **interstitial cell stimulating hormone (ICSH)** because it stimulates the secretion of testosterone by the interstitial (Leydig) cells† of the testis. FSH and LH are collectively termed the **gonadotrophins.**

6. **Prolactin** stimulates the growth and function of the mammary gland. Several other actions of prolactin are known, but their significance in human physiology is uncertain.

---

* Enrico Sertoli (1842–1910), an Italian experimental physiologist, described cells in the seminiferous tubules that are now known to be essential for the maturation of spermatozoa, a process for which testosterone is needed.

† Franz von Leydig (1821–1908) was a German comparative histologist.

Releasing and Inhibiting Hormones

The neurons that produce the substances released into the hypophysial portal vessels have their somata in the tuber cinereum and in the anterior hypothalamic and preoptic areas. The unmyelinated axons of these cells end on the blood vessels of the median eminence. The nuclei that project to the median eminence are collectively called the **hypophysiotropic area.**

The following releasing and inhibitory hormones (or factors) are well known. All except dopamine are peptides, and most of them also occur in neurons in other parts of the central and peripheral nervous systems. Each hormone's release from the anterior lobe is controlled mainly by its releasing factor except prolactin, the release of which is restrained by dopamine.

1. **Corticotrophin releasing hormone** (CRH)
2. **Thyrotropin releasing hormone** (TRH)
3. **Growth hormone releasing hormone** (GRH or SRH)
4. **Somatostatin** inhibits STH release (though this may not be its normal function)
5. **Luteinizing hormone releasing hormone** (LHRH; also called gonadotrophin releasing hormone, GnRH) stimulates secretion of both FSH and LH
6. **Dopamine** inhibits the release of prolactin

The ependymal cells of the floor of the third ventricle are tanycytes (see Chap. 2). Their long basal processes end as synapselike boutons in contact with capillaries and axons in the median eminence. It has been speculated that the tanycytes convey some kind of chemical message from the cerebrosinal fluid to the hypophysis. In monkeys, the ultrastructural appearance of the tanycytes changes with the phases of the menstrual cycle.

Chapter 27

Visceral Innervation

The autonomic nervous system is described superficially in Chapter 6, which the student may wish to review. Now the anatomy of the human autonomic system is treated in more detail, together with the autonomic neurotransmitters, visceral sensory innervation, and the reflexes that control the cardiovascular and respiratory systems.

Distribution of Cranial and Spinal Preganglionic Fibers

Parasympathetic preganglionic fibers leave the brain stem in cranial nerves III, VII, IX, and X, and leave the spinal cord in nerves S2, S3, and S4. From the esophagus to the splenic flexure of the colon, the enteric nervous system receives vagal preganglionic fibers. The distal colon and rectum receive sacral preganglionic input. In addition, postganglionic sympathetic fibers end in all parts of the enteric nervous system.

Preganglionic sympathetic fibers are the axons of somata in the lateral horn of the gray matter of segments T1 to L3 of the spinal cord. These myelinated fibers leave the cord in the ventral root. Distal to the fusion of dorsal and ventral roots, the preganglionic fibers depart from the spinal nerve in the **white communicating ramus,** which passes ventrally to enter the sympathetic ganglion associated with its segmental level. The thoracic and lumbar sympathetic ganglia are on the inside of the posterior (dorsal) wall of the thorax and abdomen, outside the pleura and the peritoneum, close to the lateral surfaces of the vertebral bodies. They are called **paravertebral ganglia,** and more will be said about them in the next section of this chapter.

Having entered one of the paravertebral ganglia T1 to L3, a preganglionic axon may do one of three things (Fig. 27-1):

1. It may end there by synapsing with neurons in the ganglion.
2. It may turn rostrally or caudally in the sympathetic trunk to terminate in another ganglion. This is how preganglionic fibers reach the sympathetic ganglia of segments rostral to T1 or caudal to L3.
3. It may pass through the paravertebral ganglion without synapsing and continue in one of the splanchnic nerves.

The **splanchic nerves** are formed from preganglionic fibers that pass *through* sympathetic ganglia. The name "splanchnic" comes from the Greek for "entrails." It indicates that these nerves go to the **pre-aortic** and **pelvic sympathetic ganglia,** which supply the organs in the abdomen.

The celiac, superior mesenteric, and inferior mesenteric ganglia lie to left and right of the sites of origin of the corresponding arteries, which are unpaired branches of the aorta. The ganglia are therefore called **pre-aortic gan-**

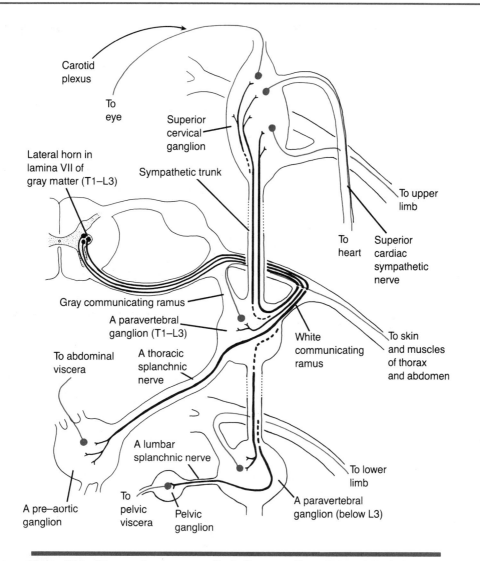

Figure 27-1 Diagram showing preganglionic fibers, ganglia, and postganglionic fibers of the sympathetic nervous system. The *adrenal medulla* (not shown) is supplied by preganglionic fibers from the lowest splanchnic nerve.

glia. Similar but smaller sympathetic ganglia are associated with the paired renal arteries. The **pelvic ganglia** (see Fig. 27-1) can be thought of as pre-aortic ganglia that are caudal to the aortic bifurcation.

Preganglionic sympathetic fibers also end in the **adrenal medulla.** The cells of the adrenal medulla are sympathetic neurons that have no axons; they secrete adrenaline and noradrenaline into the blood.

Sympathetic Ganglia and Postganglionic Fibers

Paravertebral Ganglia

There is a paravertebral ganglion for each spinal nerve. The ganglia for the eight cervical segments are fused together, however, to form three cervical sympathetic ganglia. The **superior cervical ganglion** is the largest. The inferior cervical ganglion is, in most people, fused with the sympathetic ganglion of T1 to form the **stellate ganglion.** The line of connected ganglia on each side is the **sympathetic trunk** or **chain.** The two chains join caudally at the **ganglion impar** (unpaired ganglion), anterior to the base of the coccyx.

The axons of the neurons in the paravertebral ganglia are distributed in postganglionic nerves of three kinds (see Fig. 27-1):

1. Every spinal nerve receives a **gray communicating ramus** from its sympathetic ganglion. (It is gray because postganglionic autonomic fibers are unmyelinated.) The postganglionic axons are then distributed through plexuses and nerves to muscles and skin. They supply the smooth muscle of blood vessels and of piloarrector muscles, and also the eccrine sweat glands.
2. A **cardiac sympathetic** nerve arises from each cervical sympathetic ganglion. The largest, the superior cardiac sympathetic nerve, comes from the superior cervical ganglion and then accompanies the vagus into the thorax. The sympathetic axons end in the pacemaker tissue (sinuatrial node) of the right atrium and among the ordinary cardiac muscle fibers of the ventricles.
3. The **carotid plexus** consists of postganglionic sympathetic axons that leave the superior (rostral) pole of the superior cervical ganglion and accompany the internal and external carotid arteries and their branches, providing the head with sympathetic innervation. Fibers leave the carotid plexus as follows: (a) Some go to muscles, skin, and mucous membranes; (b) others enter cranial parasympathetic ganglia, but pass through without synapsing and go to smooth muscles and glands. In the lacrimal and salivary glands, the sympathetic fibers supply blood vessels and make a minor contribution to the control of secretion. The smooth muscles supplied by sympathetic fibers are the dilator pupillae in the iris and some of the fibers of the levator palpebrae superioris. Most fibers of the latter muscle are striated and are supplied by the oculomotor nerve.

Pre-aortic and Pelvic Ganglia

The pre-aortic ganglia are close to the branches of the abdominal aorta. Their postganglionic fibers are distributed in the adventitial (outermost) layers of the walls of the arteries and their branches. Consequently the ganglia supply the same organs as the arteries. The **celiac ganglion** supplies the stomach and also sends fibers to the esophagus, liver, spleen, and pancreas. The **superior mesenteric ganglion** supplies the small intestine and the ascending and transverse colon. The **inferior mesenteric ganglion** supplies the descending colon and rectum. The **renal ganglia** supply the kidneys. The **pelvic ganglia** send axons to the blood vessels and some of the smooth musculature of the urinary and reproductive tracts and also contribute to the innervation of the rectum.

Actions of the Sympathetic System

Blood Vessels

Impulses in sympathetic axons cause *vasoconstriction in skin, mucous membranes, and abdominal viscera,* and *vasodilatation in muscles.* The mechanism for producing contraction of smooth muscle in some sites and relaxation in others is described later in this chapter, in the section concerned with neurotransmitters.

The coronary arteries, which supply the musculature of the heart, are not controlled by autonomic nerve fibers. They dilate in response to metabolites released by the contracting cardiac muscle fibers and in response to circulating adrenaline. The blood vessels of the central nervous system respond to local metabolites and to their own internal pressures (see Chap. 29).

Skin

The eccrine sweat glands and piloarrector muscles are stimulated by their sympathetic innervation.

Heart

The sinuatrial node and the ventricular myocardium are stimulated by the sympathetic system, which *accelerates the rate* of beating (chronotropic effect) and *increases the force of systolic contraction* (inotropic effect). Both actions increase the amount of work done by the heart.

Respiratory Passages

The smooth muscle in bronchioles and smaller bronchi relaxes in response to the sympathetic neurotransmitter. The diameters of the tubes are thereby increased, reducing resistance to the flow of air.

Eye

The pupil dilates when the radial fibers of the iris contract. The smooth muscle fibers in the upper eyelid help to keep the eye open.

Alimentary Canal

Sympathetic activity causes vasoconstriction and has the general effect of slowing propulsion along the gastrointestinal tract. The sphincters contract, and the ordinary smooth muscle relaxes.

Reproductive System

The ductus deferens (= vas deferens) is supplied with sympathetic fibers. These cause peristaltic movements that carry spermatozoa from the epididymis to the urethra. (The ejaculation of semen from the urethra is effected largely by contractions of the bulbospongiosus, a striated skeletal muscle.)

Adrenal Medulla

The modified sympathetic neurons that are the endocrine cells of the adrenal medulla secrete their hormones into the blood. These hormones (especially adrenaline) act upon the liver to promote the mobilization of glucose from stored glycogen, thereby increasing the concentration of glucose in the blood. Circulating adrenaline also causes dilatation of the coronary vessels and secretion from the apocrine sweat glands in the armpits and elsewhere. Bilateral removal of the adrenal medulla does not result in disability. (The adrenal cortex, by contrast, is essential for life.)

Some Disorders of the Sympathetic Nervous System

The most conspicuous effects of loss of sympathetic control are seen in the eye and the skin. The preganglionic fibers that supply the dilator pupillae, the smooth muscle of the eyelid, and the skin of the face enter the stellate ganglion and turn rostrally to end in the superior cervical ganglion. A destructive lesion of the sympathetic chain at or rostral to the stellate ganglion causes **Horner's syndrome** (named after Johann Horner, 1831–1886, a Swiss ophthalmologist). The syndrome consists of constriction of the pupil with drooping (not closure) of the upper eyelid. The affected eye also appears to be retracted into the orbit. Careful observation reveals other abnormalities: loss of sweating, vasomotor control, and piloarrection on the affected side of the face.

Horner's syndrome can occur, ipsilaterally, in the lateral medullary syndrome (see Chap. 15). The sympathetic dysfunction is probably due to transection of hypothalamo-spinal, hypothalamo-reticular, or reticulospinal pathways.

Surgical sympathectomy increases the blood flow through the sympathetically denervated skin, but does not improve the vascular perfusion of muscles. The operation was once fashionable as a treatment for peripheral vascular disease, but is now rarely done.

Cranial Parasympathetic System

The parasympathetic components of the cranial nerves are reviewed and illustrated in Chapters 19 and 20. Their functions are as follows.

Oculomotor Nerve

The preganglionic axons end in the ciliary ganglion, which supplies the sphincter pupillae and ciliary muscles.

Pupillary dilatation is the earliest sign of compression of the oculomotor nerve. At first the light reflex is less brisk than on the normal side. Eventually the pupil is widely dilated and unresponsive. The commonest cause is a subdural hemorrhage (see Chap. 28).

Facial and Glossopharyngeal Nerves

The lacrimal and salivatory nuclei contain the somata of the preganglionic fibers. The parasympathetic ganglia are: (a) The pterygopalatine ganglion, which supplies the lacrimal and nasal glands: (b) the submandibular ganglion, which supplies the submandibular and sublingual glands; and (c) the otic ganglion, which supplies the parotid gland. The parasympathetic innervation is the principal mechanism stimulating production of saliva, tears, and the secretions of the nose and paranasal sinuses.

Vagus Nerve

The nucleus ambiguus contains cells whose axons end in the tiny cardiac ganglia around the roots of the great vessels. Postganglionic fibers supply the nodal (pacemaker) muscle fibers of the right atrium and the musculature of the atria and ventricles. Activity of the parasympathetic supply *makes the heart beat more slowly and reduces the force of contraction.*

The dorsal nucleus of the vagus contains preganglionic neurons whose axons end within the enteric neurons system, from the esophagus to the splenic flexure of the colon. Parasympathetic activity *increases propulsive movements* in the alimentary canal and causes *relaxation of sphincters. Secretion* from glands, notably of acid and pepsin in the stomach, is stimulated. Vagal fibers also end in ganglia that send secretomotor fibers to the *pancreas* and the *bronchi.*

Sacral Parasympathetic System

The preganglionic axons leave the cord in the ventral roots of nerves S2 to S4 and are distributed to small parasympathetic ganglia within a plexus of nerves that surrounds the pelvic viscera. Postganglionic axons go to various organs:

1. The enteric nervous system of the **descending colon and rectum**
2. The **detrusor** (emptying) muscle, which forms the thickest layer of the wall of the urinary bladder
3. The arteries supplying the **erectile tissue** of the penis or clitoris. The name *nervi erigentes* is often applied to the sacral preganglionic nerves

Enteric Nervous System

The enteric ganglia are disposed in two layers. The **myenteric plexus,** also named after the German anatomist Leopold Auerbach (1828–1897), is between the longitudinal and circular smooth muscle layers. The **submucous plexus,** which is commonly named after another German anatomist, Georg Meissner (1829–1905), lies in the submucosa. Tracts of nerve fibers connect the ganglia within each plexus and through the circular muscle layer. Smaller bundles of axons enter the smooth muscle and glandular tissues of the gut.

The enteric ganglia contain multipolar, bipolar, and unipolar neurons, all with unmyelinated axons. The neuroglial cells of the enteric nervous system are distinctive in that they resemble astrocytes more than Schwann cells. Nevertheless, the system is peripheral, being derived from the neural crest. The connections of the enteric neurons are summarized in Figure 27-2.

Although the extrinsic innervation of the gut is necessary for normal function, the intrinsic nervous system allows an isolated piece of intestine to make propulsive movements. These involve coordinated contraction and relaxation of the muscle fibers, which are supplied by both excitatory and inhibitory neurons. The enteric nervous system enables a large system of organs to be controlled by relatively few neurons in the central nervous system. Within the layers of smooth muscle, the responses to neurotransmitters are rapidly propagated by electrical coupling through gap junctions that connect adjacent cells.

Partial absence of the enteric plexuses has serious consequences. **Congenital megacolon** or Hirschsprung's disease (after the Danish physician Harald Hirschsprung, 1830–1916) is a disease of infancy in which there are no myenteric or submucous ganglia in the last part of the colon and the rectum. Feces cannot be moved through this region, and there is considerable dilatation above it. The condition is cured by removal of the aganglionic segment. **South American trypanosomiasis,** commonly called Chagas' disease (Carlos Chagas, 1879–1934, was a Brazilian physician), is an

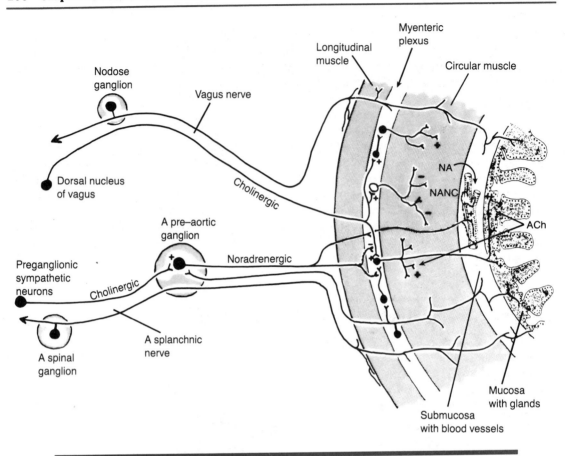

Figure 27-2   Some connections and functions of the enteric nervous system. The *submucous plexus* has been omitted for simplification. Primary sensory neurons are all shown as unipolar cells, although some of those in the gut are multipolar. *Abbreviations:* **+** = Excitatory. **−** = Inhibitory. **ACh** = Acetylcholine. **NA** = Noradrenaline. **NANC** = Nonadrenergic, noncholinergic transmission, which is inhibitory to the smooth muscle.

important cause of ill health in the new world tropics. One of its many complications is megaesophagus, due to loss of enteric neurons necessary for the passage of swallowed food into the stomach. The causative protozoan shares a surface antigen with enteric neurons; the latter are destroyed by immune mechanisms evoked by the infection.

Some **purgatives** work by stimulating the myenteric plexus of the colon. Excessive use of these drugs, a curious kind of addiction,

can kill the neurons. The colon then becomes incapable of propulsive movement, an outcome known as cathartic colon. Surgical removal of the colon is necessary in the most severe cases.

Neurotransmitters in the Autonomic System

The first evidence for chemical synaptic transmission was obtained with autonomically innervated organs, and the Nobel prize for Physiology or Medicine was awarded in 1936 to Otto Loewi (1873–1961), a German (later American) physiologist who demonstrated the chemical nature of neural transmission to the heart, and to H.H. Dale (1875–1969), the English pharmacologist and physiologist who introduced the terms "cholinergic" and "adrenergic." Both words are still used, although the latter is now usually rendered as "noradrenergic." (Truly adrenergic neurons, which use adrenaline as their transmitter, occur in the brain stem but not in the peripheral autonomic system.)

Acetylcholine

Acetylcholine (ACh) is the transmitter used by *all preganglionic neurons,* whether of the sympathetic system or parasympathetic system, and also by *all postganglionic parasympathetic neurons* and by the *sympathetic neurons that supply eccrine sweat glands.* Those enteric neurons that are excitatory to smooth muscle and glands are also cholinergic. Two types of receptors occur on cells that receive cholinergic innervation. **Nicotinic receptors,** so named because they can be stimulated by small doses of nicotine, are present on the neurons of autonomic ganglia. Large doses of nicotine inhibit synaptic transmission in the ganglia. **Muscarinic receptors** are present on the contractile and secretory cells innervated by cholinergic neurons of autonomic ganglia. These cells do not respond to nicotine, but they do respond to other alkaloids, of which muscarine was the first to be studied.

Drugs that competitively inhibit the action of ACh upon muscarinic receptors have various medical uses. For example, *atropine* is used by anesthetists to dry up salivary and bronchial secretions. *Hyoscine* (also called

scopolamine) is similar, but is also a sedative. *Homatropine, lachesine,* and *tropicamide* have shorter duration of action than atropine, and are used in eye drops to dilate the pupil and give the ophthalmologist a better view of the inside of the eye. Drugs that stimulate muscarinic receptors are also useful. For example *pilocarpine* is used in eye drops to constrict the pupil. *Carbachol* is sometimes used to stimulate emptying of the bladder.

Antagonists of ACh at nicotinic receptors (ganglion blockers) were used to treat high arterial blood pressure, but are now obsolete.

Noradrenaline

Noradrenaline (NA) is the transmitter used by *all neurons of sympathetic ganglia except the ones that supply eccrine sweat glands.* Various types of receptors are recognized on the surfaces of cells innervated by noradrenergic axons. The following account is greatly simplified. The **alpha receptors** are on the smooth muscle cells of blood vessels in the skin and internal organs, and on those enteric neurons that cause closure of sphincters. The dilator pupillae muscle also has alpha receptors. The **beta receptors** are those on cardiac muscle cells (pacemaker and ventricles), smooth muscle in bronchioles, small arteries in striated skeletal muscle, and enteric neurons that inhibit propulsive motility of the alimentary tract.

Several important drugs interact with noradrenergic transmission. *Noradrenaline* itself and *metaraminol* stimulate the alpha receptors strongly. They can be infused intravenously to raise the arterial blood pressure, although this procedure is no longer considered beneficial in the treatment of circulatory shock. *Isoprenaline* has stronger effects on beta receptors, so it can be used to accelerate the heart and dilate the bronchioles. There are also "beta₂-agonists" with more selective action on bronchial muscle. Such drugs include *salbutamol* and *terbutaline,* which relieve the bronchoconstriction in asthma without also stimulating the heart. *Adrenaline* stimulates alpha and beta receptors equally. It can be used to dilate the bronchioles, raise the blood pressure, and reduce blood flow through skin and mucous membranes, all at the same time, in certain allergic emergencies such as anaphylactic shock.

Antagonists acting at the alpha receptors, such as *indoramin* and *phenoxybenzamine,* are sometimes used to improve cutaneous blood flow. Numerous "beta blockers" are in clinical use. *Propranolol* is the prototype of this class of drugs. It makes the heart do less work, a desirable effect if the coronary arteries cannot deliver enough blood. Beta blockers have many other uses too.

Other Transmitters

Several peptides occur in postganglionic autonomic neurons, but their physiological functions are not yet known. The "nonadrenergic noncholinergic" (**NANC**) neurons of the enteric nervous system have been much studied. Their transmitter may be adenosine triphosphate (ATP) or vasoactive intestinal polypeptide (VIP). The NANC neurons provide inhibitory innervation to the intestinal musculature. VIP may also be involved, together with ACh, in parasympathetically mediated vasodilatation in the erectile tissue of the genitalia.

Both sympathetic and parasympathetic ganglia contain small interneurons (many with few or no neurites) that use dopamine (DA) as their transmitter. These interneurons are excited by the preganglionic axons and they may also be influenced by substances from the blood. DA inhibits the principal cells of the ganglion. The functional importance of the dopaminergic interneurons is unknown.

Sensation from Internal Organs

Viscera receive two kinds of sensory axon. Pain fibers respond to harmful stimuli. Physiological afferents are for reflexes that control the functions of the organs.

Pain Fibers

The sensory axons of viscera accompany the sympathetic and parasympathetic nerves. *All fibers concerned with visceral pain are anatomically associated with the sympathetic system.* The unipolar somata of the neurons are in spinal ganglia T1 to L3, and the distal branches of the axons pass through the white communicating rami, sympathetic ganglia, and splanchnic nerves to reach the organs of the thorax and abdomen. The central branches of the axons enter the dorsal horn of the spinal gray matter.

Visceral pain cannot usually be localized precisely and is often felt in a different part of the body. The latter phenomenon, which is of great importance in medical diagnosis, is called **referred pain.** The probable mechanism is convergence of afferent pathways from different sources in both the spinal gray matter and the thalamus. Because of the convergence, the cerebral cortex is deceived. Viscera can also give rise to accurately localized pain, which enters the spinal cord through somatic sensory nerves. This happens when a diseased organ irritates the parietal layer of the pleura or peritoneum. These membranes receive sensory innervation from the nerves that supply the abdominal and thoracic walls.

The following common examples illustrate

the principles of referral and the involvement of somatic nerves.

Pain from the **heart** is most often felt behind the sternum and in the medial side of the left arm. This pain is of the referred type, because the sensory fibers in the cardiac sympathetic nerves have their somata in the ganglia of the first five thoracic nerves.

Appendicitis begins with poorly localized pain in the center of the abdomen. When the inflamed appendix impinges on the parietal peritoneum, it does so in the territory of the 12th thoracoabdominal (intercostal) nerve, so the pain moves to the lower right corner of the abdomen and becomes sharply localized and more severe.

Referral of pain can also occur between structures innervated only by somatic nerves. For example, **toothache** is often felt in the wrong tooth or in the face or ear. Pain from an infected **paranasal sinus** is referred to the face or scalp. The parietal pleura and peritoneum covering the **diaphragm** are supplied by fibers of the phrenic nerve with sensory somata in the ganglia of C3, C4, and C5. Any pathological event impinging on the diaphragm from above or below is therefore likely to cause pain in the shoulder. The top of the shoulder is in the dermatome of C4.

Physiological Afferents for Cardiovascular and Respiratory Reflexes

Sensory fibers that modulate the cardiovascular and respiratory systems travel in cranial nerves IX and X, having their unipolar cell-bodies in the glossopharyngeal and inferior vagal (nodose) ganglia. The central branches of the axons enter the medulla and terminate in the caudal part of the **solitary nucleus.** Peripheral receptors include the **baroreceptors** (carotid sinus, aortic sinus), the **chemorecep-**

tors (carotid body, aortic body), the **volume receptors** in the atria of the heart, and the **stretch receptors** of the lungs. The solitary nucleus thus receives signals that monitor the arterial pressure, the oxygenation of the blood, the venous return to the heart, and the expansion of the lungs. Neurons in the solitary nucleus project rostrally to the hypothalamus and caudally to the preganglionic autonomic neurons of the medulla and spinal cord. The function of the carotid and aortic bodies (measurement of oxygen concentration) is supplemented by a group of **chemosensitive neurons** in the ventral part of the medullary reticular formation. These respond to changes in the pH of the cerebrospinal fluid. Such changes are ordinarily secondary to fluctuations in the concentration of carbon dioxide in the blood.

The various "vital centers" in the medulla and pons are known from physiological studies in animals. They are regions containing dendrites, somata, and axons, and they cannot all be correlated with anatomically identified nuclei in the human brain. Their principal connections and functions are as follows.

1. The **inspiratory center** is in or near the solitary nucleus. Its activity stimulates, contralaterally, the motor neurons of muscle fibers the contraction of which causes inspiration: The diaphragm (C3–C5) and the external intercostal muscles (T1–T12).

2. The **expiratory center,** near the nucleus ambiguus, is probably not involved in normal breathing. It can cause stimulation of contralateral motor neurons that supply muscles used for forced expiration: Internal intercostals, abdominal wall, and muscles connecting the spine with the shoulder girdle and ribs.

3. The **pneumotaxic center** is in or near the parabrachial nucleus in the pons. It can control the rate of respiration, perhaps by

inhibiting the inspiratory center in the medulla.

4. The **vasomotor center** in the medullary reticular formation receives afferent fibers from the solitary nucleus and projects to preganglionic sympathetic neurons in the spinal cord. These project to postganglionic neurons that supply small arteries. The calibers of small arteries are a major factor determining the pressure in the larger arteries. Pressor and depressor regions of the vasomotor center are recognized.

5. Among central connections controlling the **heart rate** are those from the solitary nucleus to the nucleus ambiguus. These nuclei, as well as the preganglionic sympathetic neurons in the upper thoracic segments of the cord, are influenced by input from the hypothalamus and reticular formation.

Pelvic Visceral Reflexes

The emptying of bowel and bladder in man are voluntary acts that modulate the autonomic nervous system. These functions can occur reflexively, however, in response to filling, in paraplegic patients. The reflexes are mediated by sensory fibers that accompany the pelvic parasympathetic nerves. The synapses are in the sacral spinal gray matter. Erection of the penis and ejaculation of semen can also be achieved by paraplegic men in response to tactile stimulation. The transected spinal cord prevents conscious sensory perception of these events.

Chapter 28

Ensheathment

of the Nervous System

Neurons and neuroglial cells are not physically strong. It is therefore necessary for the cells of nervous tissue to be braced by stronger elements. Such protection is provided by the axial skeleton and by special layers of connective tissue that form the sheaths of peripheral nerves and the meninges of the central nervous system. The name **"meninges"** (singular, "meninx") is from the Greek for "membranes").

Sheaths of Peripheral Nerves and Ganglia

The structure of a **nerve** is best appreciated in a transverse section (Fig. 28-1). The axons and neuroglia (Schwann cells) are gathered into small bundles, the **fascicles.** Each fascicle is surrounded by several layers of flattened cells, which constitute the **perineurium.** The territory inside the perineurium is the **endoneurium.** In addition to nerve fibers, the endoneurium contains capillary blood vessels and connective tissue.

Outside the perineurium is the **epineurium,** which consists of the connective tissue intervening between fascicles and surrounding the whole nerve. The epineurium contains many collagen fibers and accounts for the nerve's tensile strength and resistance to buffeting by nearby bones, muscles, or skin.

In spinal and autonomic ganglia, the neurons and satellite cells are surrounded by ordinary collagenous connective tissue similar to that of the epineurium. Within the cranial cavity and spinal canal, the epineurium is lacking, so the nerve roots are thinner and more fragile than ordinary nerves.

Meninges

In fishes and amphibians, a single layer of connective tissue called the primitive meninx intervenes between the central nervous system and the cartilage or bone of the skull and spinal canal. In mammals there are three layers.

The Leptomeninges

The leptomeninges ("thin membranes") are two layers of cellular connective tissue separated by a space. In embryonic development a single layer, derived at least in part from the neural crest, first ensheaths the whole central nervous system. Extracellular spaces then develop within the single layer. When the spaces have become confluent, there are

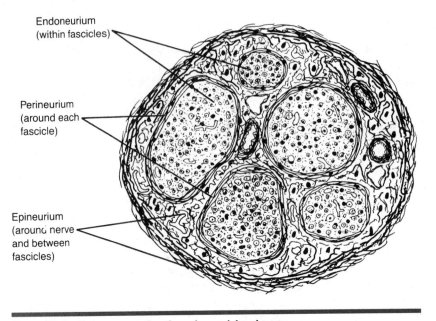

Endoneurium
(within fascicles)

Perineurium
(around each
fascicle)

Epineurium
(around nerve
and between
fascicles)

Figure 28-1   Transverse section through a peripheral nerve.

separate outer and inner layers joined by delicate strands (trabeculae) that form bridges across the intervening space. The outer leptomeninx contains no blood vessels. It is called the **arachnoid.** This name comes from the Greek for a spider's web, to which the membrane bears some resemblance. The inner leptomeningeal layer, which contains many blood vessels, is the **pia mater** (Latin for "tender mother"). The pia mater and arachnoid are collectively called the **pia-arachnoid.** The two layers are reflected upon the surfaces of blood vessels that transverse the intervening subarachnoid space.

The pia mater is only a few cells thick and is closely applied to the surface of the brain and spinal cord, following the contours of every crevice and convolution. The arachnoid is applied to the inside of the dura mater, which is described below. Because the dura lines the cranial cavity, the arachnoid does not conform to the surface of the brain. Con-

sequently the **subarachnoid space** is widest over concavities such as sulci and narrowest over convexities such as gyri (see Fig. 28-2). The subarachnoid space is completely filled with **cerebrospinal fluid (CSF),** which forms a liquid cushion between the central nervous system and the axial skeleton. The blending of the pia-arachnoid with the outside surfaces of arteries and veins ensures that as these vessels enter the brain they are surrounded by spaces containing CSF. The spaces are present around arterioles and venules, but not around capillaries (except in the circumventricular organs; see Chap. 30).

Meningitis is inflammation of the meninges, usually due to infection by bacteria. Most types of meningitis are due to proliferation of the offending organisms in the CSF, with a consequent inflammatory reaction of the blood vessels of the pia mater. Proteins and leukocytes enter the CSF through the walls of the reactive blood vessels, and the surface

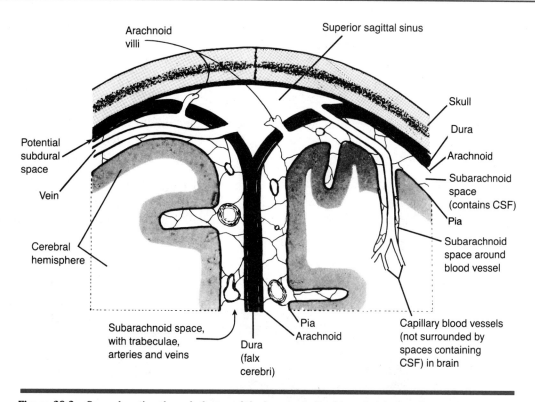

Figure 28-2 Coronal section through the top of the human skull, with underlying meninges, blood vessels, and brain. Two veins in the subarachnoid space are shown entering a dural venous sinus. Two arachnoid villi (see Chap. 30) are also shown.

of the brain may be locally irritated or injured by the production of pus. This can cause functional abnormality appropriate to the site of the insult. The most conspicuous symptoms of meningitis, however, are fever and pain in the head and neck. The pain results from stimulation of pain-sensitive axons in the dura, which is next to the arachnoid.

Infections that spread slowly can cause less spectacular forms of meningitis. The slowly growing lesions of tuberculosis or syphilis, for example, can cause a great variety of symptoms from interference either with the nervous system directly or with the circulation of cerebrospinal fluid.

The Dura Mater

This membrane is nearly always called the **dura.** The name *dura mater* in Latin means "hard mother." It is occasionally called the "pachymeninx," from the Greek for "thick membrane." The dura is rich in collagen. Inside the skull it adheres tightly to the bone except where there are spaces, filled with venous blood, between the dura and the periosteum. These spaces, the **dural venous sinuses,** receive the veins that drain the brain. After flowing through the sinuses, the blood leaves the skull by way of the internal jugular vein.

The structure of a dural venous sinus is best appreciated in a transverse section such as Figure 28-2. This diagram also illustrates the pia-arachnoid and the arachnoid villi, through which CSF is absorbed into the blood (see Chap. 30).

Where a sinus is formed, the dural membranes may continue to project into the cranial cavity as a **dural reflection.** This is a membrane that intervenes between two major parts of the brain. The largest dural reflections are the **falx cerebri,** between the cerebral hemispheres, and the **tentorium cerebelli** sep-

arating the occpital lobes from the cerebellar hemispheres. (*Falx* is the Latin for "sickle," *tentorium* for "tent." Both terms reasonably describe the shapes of the dural reflections.) The straight sinus is formed where the falx and the tentorium meet, so all its walls are made of reflected dura.

The positions of the major venous sinuses and dural reflections are shown in Figure 28-3.

The dura mater of the cranium is continuous at the foramen magnum with that of the spinal canal. The **spinal dura** is not adherent

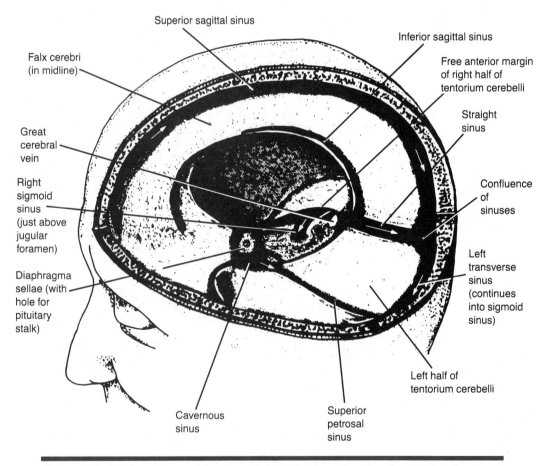

Figure 28-3   Interior of the cranial cavity with the brain removed to show dural folds and venous sinuses. White arrows indicate direction of flow of blood.

to the walls of the canal, but is surrounded by fatty connective tissue containing a plexus of veins. Caudally, the dura ends within the sacrum. Caudal to that level, the bony canal contains fat, veins, the roots of the coccygeal and last three sacral nerves, and the **filum terminale.** The last-named structure is a filament of neuroglial tissue connecting the caudal tip of the spinal cord with the coccyx. It is the vestige of the spinal cord of the tail, which regresses in embryonic development.

Where a nerve leaves the skull or spinal canal through a foramen, the dura blends with the epineurium. The arachnoid is continuous with the perineurium, and the pia mater is continuous with the endoneurial connective tissue. In the nerve roots, there is continuity between the subarachnoid space and the extracellular space of the endoneurium.

Local anesthetic drugs can be injected into the extradural space of the caudal end of the spinal canal to cause loss of the sensation mediated by the sacral segmental nerves. This procedure, known as **epidural anesthesia,** is much used in obstetrics. With **spinal anesthesia,** the drug is injected into the subarachnoid space caudal to the spinal cord. The rostral limit of the anesthetized region is determined by the volume injected and by the patient's posture.

Meningeal Sensation

The leptomeninges do not contain sensory nerve fibers, but the dura is abundantly furnished with pain-sensitive axons. Most of the cranial dura is supplied by branches of the trigeminal nerve. That lining the occipital region receives fibers from the vagus nerve and spinal nerves C2 and C3 (also C1 in individuals in whom C1 has a dorsal root). The spinal dura receives branches from all the spinal nerves.

The pain in any kind of meningitis is due to irritation of the dura. Associated rigidity of the neck is a defensive reflex initiated by attempting to move the cervical spinal dura. Another clinical sign of meningeal irritation is reflex muscular resistance to an attempt to straighten the knee when the hip is flexed. This movement pulls on the sciatic nerve, which pulls, in turn, on the spinal dura.

Intracranial Hemorrhages

Bleeding within the cranial cavity is always a serious event. The skull cannot stretch to accomodate the blood, so the nervous tissue is pressed upon.

Extradural Hemorrhage

A blow to the side of the head can crack the thin squamous part of the temporal bone and damage the **middle meningeal artery.** This vessel is in the periosteum. When it bleeds the released blood forces the dura away from the skull, forming an intracranial mass that presses on the cerebral hemisphere. The hemorrhage, being arterial, is quite rapid, so clinical signs develop quickly. They are similar to those of subdural hemorrhage.

Subdural Hemorrhage

With most head injuries, there is sudden rotational acceleration and deceleration of the head. The brain is a substantial mass suspended weightlessly in the cerebrospinal fluid. It is tethered to the vault of the skull only by superficial cerebral veins, which enter the superior sagittal sinus. Violent movement of the brain inside the subarachnoid space can tear one of the fragile veins at the place where it pierces the dura. The hemorrhage is typically slow, because the pressure in the CSF is higher than that in the dural venous sinuses. The blood clots as it accumulates between the dura and the arachnoid, forming a **subdural**

hematoma. This mass presses upon the cerebral hemisphere.

As a result of pressure from above, *the cerebral hemisphere is pushed downwards into the notch in the anterior margin of the tenorium cerebelli.* There is progressive deterioration of consciousness, associated with signs of increasing damage to the oculomotor nerve (see Chap. 19), which is stretched over the free anterior margin of the tentorium. The first fibers to be affected are the preganglionic parasympathetic axons, which lie near the surface of the nerve. The pupillary light reflex becomes sluggish and is then lost. Eventually the pupil is widely dilated. The oculomotor nerve on the side of the hematoma is the one more commonly affected. Sometimes the one-sided pressure from above presses the opposite side of the midbrain against the tentorial notch, injuring corticospinal, corticopontine, and corticoreticular fibers in the ventral part of the cerebral peduncle. In such cases, the contralateral oculomotor nerve is stretched. The result is a hemiplegia on the same side as the hematoma, with paralysis of the contralateral oculomotor nerve. In fatal cases of subdural hematoma, a groove in the uncus shows the pathologist where the medial part of the temporal lobe was forced into the tentorial notch.

Subdural hemorrhages are not always easily diagnosed, because the delay before the onset of symptoms may vary from nothing to several weeks. It is nonetheless essential to detect the condition, because surgical evacuation of the hematoma is usually curative.

Tentorial herniation may also be caused by masses other than subdural hematomas, such as tumors or abscesses of the cerebrum. *The presence of raised intracranial pressure, indicated by papilloedema (see Chap. 30) contraindicates withdrawal of cerebrospinal fluid from the lumbar cistern.* A lumbar puncture (spinal tap) is likely to cause herniation by producing a rostrocaudal gradient of pressure. The worst outcome is **medullary coning,** which occurs when the medulla and the tonsils of the cerebellum are forced into the foramen magnum, causing coma and death from compression of the medulla.

Subarachnoid Hemorrhage

Bleeding into the subarachnoid space may come from an aneurysm of one of the arteries at the base of the brain or from a tumor containing fragile blood vessels. An aneurysm is a bulge due to weakness of the wall of an artery. Typically there is a severe headache of sudden onset, with vomiting and the signs of meningeal irritation. Coma and death may follow if the hemorrhage is a large one. Aneurysms are sometimes amenable to surgical treatment, which can remove the risk of a subsequent fatal hemorrhage.

Cerebral Hemorrhage

The most common cause of bleeding within the brain is rupture of a microscopic aneurysm at the base of the cerebral hemisphere. Such aneurysms occur in patients with high arterial blood pressure (hypertension). Successful control of hypertension by drugs has greatly reduced the incidence of cerebral hemorrhage. The escaping blood damages white and gray matter, causing hemiplegia, often followed by coma and death. Signs of tentorial herniation or of blood in the subarachnoid space may also be present.

Hemorrhage can occur in other parts of the brain, including the pons and the cerebellum. A large **pontine hemorrhage** causes instant death, but a smaller lesion may cause the "locked in" syndrome (see Chap. 21). **Cerebellar hemorrhages** are rare and difficult to diagnose, but the patient's life can sometimes by saved by prompt surgical intervention. Signs of rapidly increasing intracranial pressure (Chap. 30) are associated with those of cerebellar dysfunction.

Chapter 29

Blood Vessels

of the Central

Nervous System

The brain and spinal cord receive about one fifth of the oxygenated blood pumped out by the heart. The total flow does not vary much with activity, although there are functionally related changes in blood flow through specific regions. Inadequate supply of oxygen by arteries is the cause of **stroke,** one of the most common disorders of the human nervous system.

Local cerebral blood flow is studied by plotting the distribution of radioactively labelled blood. Regional variations in glucose utilization can be similarly examined, using labelled 2-deoxyglucose. This compound is taken up by cells as if it were glucose, but it is not consumed in metabolic processes.

Arteries of the Brain

The brain is supplied by branches of the **internal carotid arteries** and of the **vertebral arteries.** The latter, which originate from the subclavian arteries in the base of the neck, also contribute to the vasculature of the spinal cord.

The ring of anastomosing arteries at the base of the brain is called the **circle of Willis,** after the English physician and scientist Thomas Willis (1621–1675). The origins of the arteries supplying the brain are shown in Figure 29-1. The pattern shown is variable, however. For example, one of the posterior cerebral arteries is often a branch of the internal carotid, and the diameters of the communicating arteries vary considerably among individuals.

The parts of the cerebral hemisphere supplied by the three cerebral arteries are shown in Figure 29-2. *The reader should compare this figure with the functional cortical areas delineated in Chapter 22 (see Fig. 22-3).* The territories supplied by the other arteries of the brain can be inferred from Figure 29-1. It should be noted that the anterior choroidal artery, the recurrent branch of the anterior cerebral artery, and the ganglionic arteries supply most of the interior of the cerebral hemisphere and diencephalon. The posterior inferior cerebellar artery supplies the lateral part of the medulla, a region of greater functional importance than the posterior and inferior regions of the cerebellum.

The arteries forming the circle of Willis can dilate if one of the vessels feeding the circle

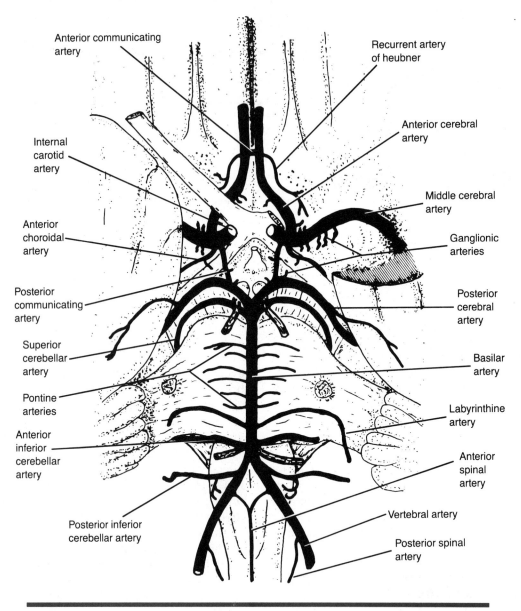

Figure 29-1   Arteries on the ventral surface of the brain.

is slowly occluded. The anastomoses cannot usually cope with a sudden arterial blockage. There are limited anastomoses between arterial branches on the surface of the brain, but none in the interior.

Venous Drainage of the Brain

Some of the veins of the brain are illustrated in Figure 29-3. Anastomoses ensure that venous occlusion is not serious, except on the

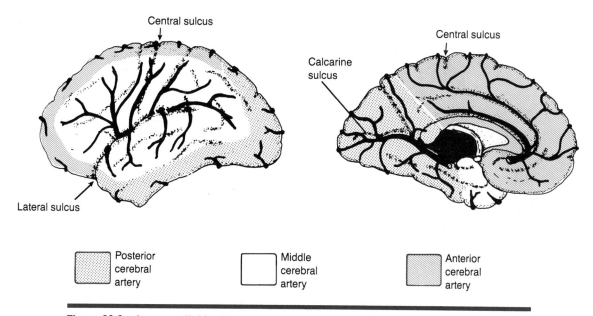

Figure 29-2 Areas supplied by the three cerebral arteries. This figure should be compared with Figure 22-3, which shows the functional areas of the cortex.

rare occasions when the dural venous sinuses are blocked. Subdural hemorrhage from the superficial cerebral veins, a common complication of head injury, is described in Chapter 28.

Blood Supply of the Spinal Cord

The **anterior spinal artery,** a median vessel, and the paired **posterior spinal arteries** are branches of the vertebral arteries. All three vessels are small, but they anastomose along the length of the cord with **radicular arteries,** which enter the spinal canal alongside the segmental nerve roots.

Anterior and posterior **spinal veins,** which accompany the arteries, drain into radicular veins. The latter vessels drain into the venous plexus of the epidural space, from which the blood is eventually conducted into the vertebral, intercostal, and lumbar veins.

The spinal cord is easily damaged, with consequent paraplegia, by obstruction of its arteries (causing ischaemia) or its veins (causing swelling and resultant pressure).

Cerebral Vascular Disease

Blood vessels can cause trouble either by leaking or by being blocked. Various kinds of intracranial hemorrhage are discussed in Chapter 28. Arterial obstruction, which may be due to thrombosis or embolism,* is consid-

---

* *Thrombosis* occurs when a *thrombus* forms in an artery or vein, or in the heart. A thrombus is a mass of platelets and coagulated blood, produced when the endothelial lining of a blood vessel or of the heart is diseased. The most common cause of thrombosis is *atheroma,* also called *arteriosclerosis,* in which fatty material accumulates in the walls of arteries. Venous thrombosis can be due to nearby inflammation, injury, or obstruction. *Embolism* occurs when a thrombus is set free in the circulating blood. A venous thrombus will lodge in

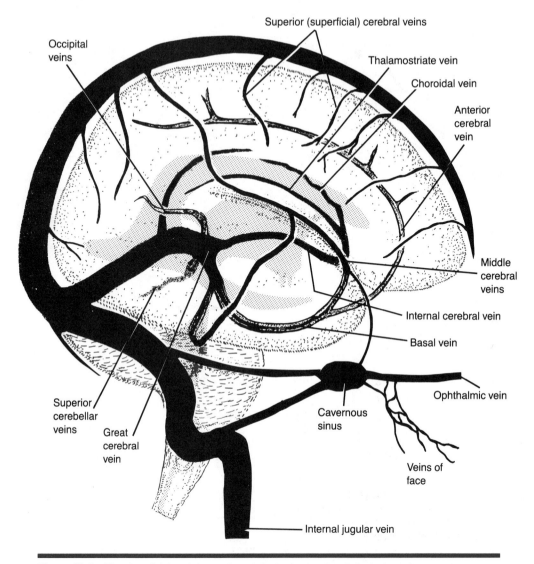

Figure 29-3   The superficial and deep veins of the brain showing their drainage into the dural venous sinuses. The surface of the brain and the outline of the ventricular system are shown in color.

ered here, and some effects of venous thrombosis are also described.

the pulmonary arterial circulation. A thrombus from the left atrium will end up blocking a systemic artery, which may be one of those supplying the brain.

Arterial Insufficiency

The consequences of obstruction of an artery depend upon the normal function of the part of the brain deprived of its blood supply. The onset of symptoms is faster with embolism than with thrombosis. When arteries are narrowed by atheroma, there may be **transient**

ischemic attacks. These are episodes of inadequate oxygenation in which the symptoms of arterial occlusion last for only a few minutes. A **stroke** is the disease caused by rapidly developing blockage of a cerebral artery, or by hemorrhage from such a vessel. The typical results of occlusion of some of the intracranial arteries are as follows:

Internal carotid artery—Contralateral hemiplegia, with sensory deficits and (if the hemisphere dominant for speech is involved) aphasia. A thrombus or embolus is often surgically accessible.

Middle cerebral artery—Effects are similar to those of internal carotid occlusion, but obstruction of branches of the middle cerebral artery can lead to defective function of smaller areas. The cortical areas for the lower limb are spared.

Anterior cerebral artery—If its recurrent branch, the artery of Heubner, is involved, there is contralateral hemiplegia, including paralysis of the lower half of the face. Heubner's artery, described by the German pediatrician Johann Heubner (1843–1926), supplies part of the internal capsule. Obstruction distal to the origin of Heubner's artery causes paralysis and sensory insufficiency only in the lower limb.

Posterior cerebral artery—There is blindness in the contralateral visual fields of both eyes, and sometimes loss of pursuit movement of the eyes to the contralateral side, although saccadic movements are unaffected (see Chap. 19). There may also be visual agnosia.

Basilar artery—Complete occlusion is usually fatal. Transient failure of circulation through the ventral part of the brain stem can be due to occlusion of one subclavian artery, proximal to the origin of the vertebral artery. Blood from the normal subclavian artery then flows across the junction of the two vertebral arteries into the distal branches of the obstructed vessel. Consequently, blood that should go into the basilar artery is at times diverted to the upper limb. This is the *subclavian steal syndrome.* The symptoms can include double vision, facial paralysis, visual field defect (posterior cerebral artery), and vertigo (labyrinthine artery). Thrombosis of branches of the basilar artery can produce permanent abnormalities due to localized destruction of small parts of the brain stem.

Vertebral artery—Obstruction of one vertebral artery causes symptoms due to occlusion of its posterior inferior cerebellar branch. The lesion is illustrated in Chapter 15 (see Fig. 15-7). There is vertigo (vestibular nuclei), difficulty swallowing (nucleus ambiguus), and ipsilateral cerebellar ataxia. There is loss of pain and temperature sensation on the same side of the face (caudal part of the spinal trigeminal nucleus) and opposite side of the body below the neck (spinal lemniscus). Involvement of (presumed) hypothalamo-reticular and reticulospinal fibers concerned with the sympathetic nervous system often produces an ipsilateral Horner's syndrome (see Chap. 27).

Diseases of Veins

Occlusion of the transverse sinus sometimes occurs aseptically as a complication of infection in the nearby middle ear. There is raised intracranial pressure but few symptoms. Thrombosis of the dural venous sinuses due to direct invasion by bacteria is a much more serious matter. Bacteria may enter the sinuses by spreading from the middle ear or the frontal sinus of the nose. The raised intracranial pressure is combined with all the features of a serious infection. Obstruction of veins entering the superior sagittal sinus can cause motor and sensory abnormalities due to inadequate circulation in the cerebral cortex.

The **cavernous sinus** receives veins from the

face and orbit. Septic thrombosis of this sinus is a result of infection spreading along tributary veins, typically from a carbuncle on the upper lip. The tissues of the orbit become greatly swollen, and there is paralysis of cranial nerves III, IV, and VI and impaired sensation from the skin supplied by the ophthalmic and maxillary divisions of V. These nerves pass through the sinus. The neurological abnormalities are added to the general effects of severe infection. The same clinical features, but without infection, are seen if the internal carotid artery leaks, through a ruptured weak spot in its walls, into the cavernous sinus. Then there is also pulsation of the protruding eyeball and a loud noise in the head that can be heard with a stethoscope. These disorders are rare, but they illustrate important points of anatomy.

Regulation of Cerebral Blood Vessels

The sympathetic nervous system does not have a significant vasomotor function in the central nervous system. The major regulatory mechanism, known as **autoregulation,** is due to an intrinsic property of the smooth muscle cells in the arteries; they contract if they are stretched by increased intraluminal pressure. Thus vasoconstriction will protect the brain if the general arterial pressure rises. Conversely dilatation of the cerebral vessels ensures adequate perfusion if there is a fall in blood pressure. Locally released metabolites, notably carbon dioxide, cause vasodilatation and may account for the locally increased blood flow observable in functionally active parts of the brain.

Blood–Brain and Blood–Nerve Barriers

Normally the neurons and neuroglial cells in most parts of the nervous system are pro-

tected from certain substances present in the circulating blood. Such substances include compounds with large molcules, notably proteins, and some with small molecules. The latter fail to enter the nervous tissue if they are bound chemically to proteins of the blood plasma. Such binding makes a small molecule behave like a large one.

Regions With and Without Blood–Tissue Barriers

The traditional method for demonstrating the blood–brain barrier is to give an animal an intravenous injection of any dye that is bound by the proteins of the plasma. The animal is killed and dissected, and it is seen that most of its organs are deeply colored. A "barrier" is present in places not colored by the dye. The most conspicuous unstained organ is the brain. There is a blood–tissue barrier in the brain, spinal cord, optic nerve, and retina. This is called the **blood–brain barrier.** The barrier is absent in a few small parts of the central nervous system, to be mentioned below. In peripheral nerves, there is a **blood–nerve barrier** within the endoneurium, but the connective tissue of the epineurium has permeable blood vessels. The diffusion of large molecules from the extracellular space of the epineurium into that of the endoneurium is prevented by the several layers of cells constituting the perineurium around each fascicle of the nerve. The perineurium itself contains no blood vessels, resembling in this respect the arachnoid with which it is continuous.

The **sites where there is no blood–brain barrier** are mostly circumventricular organs (see Chap. 30). Proteins from the blood enter the nervous tissue freely in all parts of the neurohypophysis, the epiphysis (= pineal gland), the subfornical organ, the vascular organ of the lamina terminalis, the area postrema, and the lamina cribrosa of the eye. The last-named site is where bundles of retinal axons penetrate the outer layers of the eyeball to form the optic nerve. The permeable vessels at the lamina cribrosa are probably those of the nearby choroid and sclera rather than of the central nervous tissue itself, but there is no cellular sheath to arrest the diffusion of proteins into the bundles of optic axons.

In the choroid plexuses of the brain, plasma proteins enter the extracellular space but cannot pass through the layer of choroidal ependymal cells to enter the cerebrospinal fluid. Thus there is a **blood–cerebrospinal fluid barrier,** functionally equivalent to the blood–brain barrier. Proteins introduced into the cerebrospinal fluid penetrate the ependyma and diffuse freely among the cells of the central nervous tissue; there is no cerebrospinal fluid–brain barrier.

Although a blood–nerve barrier exists in the endoneurium, there is no such barrier in sensory, sympathetic, or parasympathetic ganglia. The enteric nervous system does not contain any blood vessels. Large molecules that diffuse out of blood vessels in the intestinal muscles do not, however, enter the ganglia and tracts of the enteric nervous system. This system thus resembles the central nervous system in being shielded from plasma proteins.

Structures Forming the Barriers

The permeability of blood vessels to large molcules is studied in animals by examining tissues with the electron microscope after intravenous administration of a protein that is or can be made electron opaque. The electron micrographs reveal the sites at which the exodus of the tracer is permitted or arrested.

The capillaries of the central nervous system and of the endoneurial connective tissue of nerves have all their endothelial cells joined together by tight junctions (*zonulae occludentes*), which are impermeable to large molecules. These vessels do not have endothelial

fenestrations (holes), and any protein taken into the endothelium is returned to the lumen rather than transported across the cells. In those circumventricular organs that lack a blood–tissue barrier, the capillaries are fenestrated. This is consonant with the known or suspected endocrine or chemosensory functions of the circumventricular organs.

The capillaries of the choroid plexus are freely permeable to proteins, but these substances cannot penetrate the tight junctions that connect all adjacent choroidal ependymal cells. These cells precisely control the chemical composition of the cerebrospinal fluid, admitting only traces of proteins from the blood.

It has already been pointed out that the perineurium protects the endoneurial compartment from protein molecules that permeate from the blood into the extracellular fluid of the epineurium. The avascular arachnoid serves a similar purpose of stopping the diffusion of proteins from the dura mater, which is made of ordinary connective tissue, into the cerebrospinal fluid.

Significance of Blood–Tissue Barriers to Health and Disease

Normal Nervous Tissue

The existence of blood–brain and blood–nerve barriers suggests that most parts of the nervous system need to be protected from large molecules (and associated small molecules) that circulate in the blood. It is not obvious, however, that the lack of such protection would be harmful. When central nervous tissue from fetal animals is maintained in tissue culture, the neurons grow and form elaborate patterns of functional synaptic connections similar to those that develop in the same parts of the intact brain or spinal cord. The culture medium contains serum, the proteins of which are considered to be beneficial, not harmful. Furthermore, axons ending in muscle or connective tissue, or in regions such as the neurohypophysis that have permeable blood vessels, take up plasma proteins and transport them retrogradely. Serum albumin, for example, is normally present in the cell-bodies of motor neurons and hypothalamic neurosecretory cells.

The cerebral capillaries control the transport of inorganic ions, amino acids, and glucose into the brain, by means of pumps, channels, and carrier molecules in the membrane of the endothelial cell. Impermeability to proteins may be an incidental consequence of having blood vessels selectively permeable to smaller molecules and ions. Hydrophobic (lipid-soluble) substances that pass freely through cell membranes also cross the blood–brain interface.

Failure of the Barriers

There is often a breach in the blood–brain barrier at a site of injury or disease. The vessels around a **physical injury** are permeable to proteins for some 2 weeks after wounding. There is also abnormal permeability around sites of **infection.** In meningitis there is considerable exudation of plasma proteins into the cerebrospinal fluid. **Tumors** in the central nervous system contain and are surrounded by permeable blood vessels. This failure of the blood–brain barrier forms the basis of

gamma encephalography, which is the simplest kind of "brain scan." A compound of the radioactive element technetium (the suitably short-lived isotope [^{99}Tc]) is injected intravenously, and the head is scanned for gamma radiation. Lateral and anteroposterior pictures of the distribution of permeable blood vessels are obtained, and the position of the tumor in the brain is revealed. The method will also show a focus of inflammation such as an abscess.

The blood–brain barrier restricts the entry of many **drugs** into the central nervous system, because such substances are frequently bound to the albumin of the blood plasma. With drugs used to treat infections, impermeability usually does not matter, because the barrier is breached at the site where the drug is needed. For example, penicillin does not enter the normal brain or cerebrospinal fluid, but the antibiotic is nonetheless valuable for the treatment of bacterial meningitis.

The significance of the blood–nerve barrier is not yet understood. The endoneurial vessels become permeable distal to sites of axonal transection, and increased permeability is associated with axonal regeneration in laboratory animals. The possible functional significance of this association has been a subject of speculation by research workers interested in the reasons why cut axons can regenerate in some, but not all, parts of the nervous system (see Chap. 4).

Chapter 30

Ventricles,

Subarachnoid Space,

and Cerebrospinal Fluid

An average adult has about 140 ml of cerebrospinal fluid (**CSF**) in and around the brain and spinal cord. The fluid is continuously secreted and absorbed, at about 0.5 ml per minute. The lumen of the embryonic neural tube is obliterated in the retina, optic nerve, and olfactory bulb, so the adult ventricular system consists of the four ventricles and the central canal. The subarachnoid space forms within the developing pia-arachnoid. There is continuity from the ventricular system into the subarachnoid space through three holes in the roof of the fourth ventricle.

Ventricles and Choroid Plexuses

Lateral and Third Ventricles

Each **lateral ventricle** has the corpus callosum for its roof, the septum pellucidum and fornix for its medial wall, the thalamus for its floor, and the caudate nucleus for its lateral wall. Frontal, occipital, and temporal horns of the lateral ventricle extend into the lobes of the cerebral hemisphere. In the temporal (also called "inferior") horn, the fornix is replaced by the hippocampus. A small space between

the fornix and the anterior end of the thalamus, just behind the anterior commissure, is the **interventricular foramen,** communicating with the third ventricle.

The slitlike **third ventricle** is the space between the left and right thalami. The lower (ventral, or inferior) parts of the walls, and the floor are formed by the hypothalamus. The anterior wall of the third ventricle is the lamina terminalis, a thin layer of gray matter extending from the anterior commissure to the optic chiasma. The roof of the third ventricle is formed by the fornices of the two sides, which here are joined by commissural fibers connecting the hippocampi. Posteriorly, the third ventricle narrows into the **cerebral aqueduct,** the tubular cavity of the midbrain.

Choroid Plexus

The ventricles are lined by a simple columnar epithelium, the ependyma. This layer of cells is pushed into the cavities of the lateral and third ventricles along a line between the fornix and the thalamus by vascular connective tissue that forms the **choroid plexus** (Fig. 30-

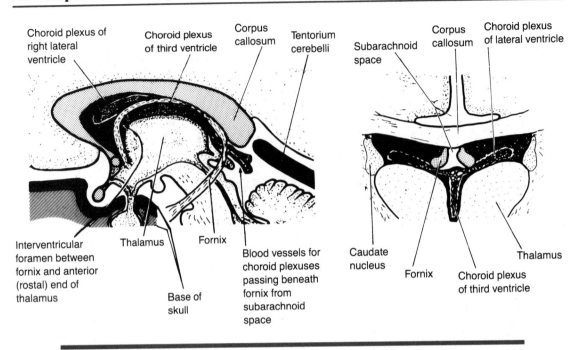

Figure 30-1 The third and lateral ventricles are shown in a dissection from the medial side (*Left*), and in coronal (transverse) section (*Right*). Shows how the choroid plexuses are invaginated from the subarachnoid space into the ventricles.

1). The ependymal cells over the surface of the choroid plexus are joined by tight junctions, so that large molecules cannot move between the cells to pass from the connective tissue into the CSF. Ordinary ependymal cells are not joined by tight junctions, and large molecules introduced into the CSF can move freely into the central nervous tissue. The capillaries of the connective tissue inside the choroid plexus have **endothelial fenestrations** (holes; from the Latin *fenestra,* a window). In this they resemble the capillaries of organs specialized for secretion (glands) or absorption (intestinal mucosa).

Fourth Ventricle

The aqueduct widens out caudally into the fourth ventricle, the cavity of the medulla and pons. This ventricle is diamond-shaped with long lateral recesses. The floor contains nuclei of cranial nerves. The four walls are the superior and inferior cerebellar peduncles. The roof of the rostral half of the fourth ventricle is a thin sheet of white matter, the **superior medullary velum,** and the fastigial nuclei of the cerebellum. The caudal half of the roof is the **inferior medullary velum,** which is a single layer of ependymal cells supported on the outside by vascular connective tissue continuous with the pia mater. The inferior velum is invaginated to form a choroid plexus similar to that of the third and lateral ventricles. Caudally, the fourth ventricle is constricted to become the **central canal** of the closed caudal part of the medulla and of the spinal cord.

There are three holes in the inferior medullary velum. The **median aperture** (foramen

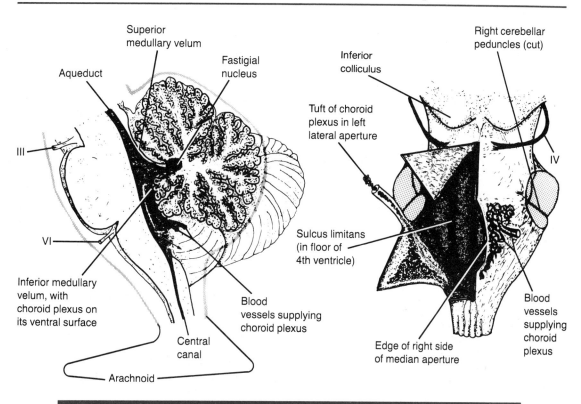

Figure 30-2   The fourth ventricle and its choroid plexus. (*Left*) A sagittal (midline) section of the brain stem, cerebellum, and associated meninges. The arrow shows the flow of cerebrospinal fluid from the fourth ventricle, through the median aperture, into the cisterna magna. (*Right*) Dorsal aspect of the brain stem after removal of the cerebellum. The roof of the fourth ventricle has been preserved on the right, but opened on the left. The tubular extension of the inferior medullary velum around the lateral aperture is really directed ventrally, not laterally, so that the tuft of choroid plexus is seen on the ventral surface (see Fig. 8-1).

of Magendie*) is in the midline. The smaller **lateral apertures** (of Luschka[†]) are at the ends of the lateral recesses (Fig. 30-2). A tuft of choroid plexus protrudes from the lateral aperture and is visible from the ventral aspect of the medulla, between the roots of cranial nerves VIII and IX. (The chemosensory neu-

rons described in Chapter 27 are close to this tuft; they monitor the concentrations of carbon dioxide in newly secreted CSF.)

Subarachnoid Space and its Cisterns

The subarachnoid space is widest where there are deep concavities in the surface of the brain. The more conspicuous enlargements are called **cisterns.** Some cisterns are important because of their anatomical relations;

---

* François Magendie (1783–1855), a French physiologist, was also one of the first (Sir Charles Bell, Chapter 20, was another) to recognize the distinct functions of dorsal and ventral roots.

[†] Hubert von Luschka (1820–1875) was a German anatomist.

others have significance as landmarks in x-rays and other images produced for clinical diagnostic purposes.

The **cerebellomedullary cistern,** or *cisterna magna,* is dorsal to the medulla and caudal (inferior) to the vermis of the cerebellum. The CSF leaving the brain by way of the median aperture enters this cistern. CSF can be sampled by a needle inserted into the cisterna magna through the back of the neck, but this is rarely done.

The **superior cistern,** above (rostral, or superior to) the midline of the cerebellum, accomodates the great cerebral vein. The term *cisterna ambiens* embrances the superior cistern and the space lateral to the midbrain.

Ventral to the brain, there are cisterns associated with the **pons,** the **interpeduncular fossa** (between the cerebral peduncles, ventral to the midbrain), the **optic chiasma,** and the **lamina terminalis.**

The top of the cranial cavity is largely filled by the cerebral hemispheres, but there is a **cistern of the lateral sulcus,** which accomodates the middle cerebral artery and veins.

The **lumbar cistern** is the largest one. It occupies the interval between the caudal end of the spinal cord (level with vertebra L2) and the caudal end of the dura (midsacral). It contains the dorsal and ventral roots of spinal nerves L3 to S5 and the filum terminale. This collection of 32 slender nerves resembles a horse's tail, hence the name *cauda equina* (from the Latin).

The subarachnoid space extends for a short distance along the roots of the spinal and cranial nerves. The arachnoid is continuous with the perineurium surrounding each fascicle in the nerve. Within the subarachnoid space, nerve roots are fragile because the epineurium is absent. This outermost sheath is acquired as the roots pierce the dura.

The **subarachnoid space around the optic nerve** is of microscopic width but great importance. It extends forward to the optic disc, where the axons of retinal ganglion cells come to-gether and traverse the choroid and sclera. (See also the account of papilledema in this chapter.)

Production and Composition of Cerebrospinal Fluid

An American pioneer of neurosurgery, Walter E. Dandy (1886–1946), discovered, in 1913, the manner of production and circulation of the cerebrospinal fluid. His experiments with animals led to conclusions that were equally applicable to man.

Production of Cerebrospinal Fluid

The most important results of the classical experiments were as follows:

1. Obstruction of one interventricular foramen caused dilatation of the lateral ventricle of the same side.
2. Obstruction of the cerebral aqueduct caused dilatation of both lateral ventricles.
3. Dilatation ceased if the obstruction was removed, or if an artificial communication was made between the ventricle and the subarachnoid space.
4. A lateral ventricle did not dilate if its choroid plexus had been removed before plugging the interventricular foramen.
5. Drops of a liquid indistinguishable from CSF were seen forming on the surface of a surgically exposed choroid plexus.

These observations leave little doubt that *the CSF is produced by the choroid plexuses, circulates through the ventricular system and enters the subarachnoid space through the apertures of the fourth ventricle.*

The way the choroid plexus works has been clarified by electron microscopy and modern physiological methods. The choroidal ependymal cells are joined by tight junctions (*zonulae occludentes*), so extracellular fluid must enter the basal poles of the cells and be secreted from their apical surfaces. There are intracellular pumps for all the common ions: Na^+, K^+, Ca^{2+}, Mg^{2+}, Cl^-, and HCO_3^-, so the ionic composition of the CSF is precisely controlled. Experiments with radioactive tracers indicate that some substances, including water, are exchanged between the CSF and both the brain tissue and the blood. Such exchange occurs throughout the ventricular system and the subarachnoid space. Nevertheless, the bulk flow of the fluid is from the choroid plexuses to the subarachnoid space, and the chemical composition of CSF is determined largely by the choroid plexuses.

Composition of Cerebrospinal Fluid

Normal CSF is blood plasma without most of the protein and with certain differences in ionic composition (Table 30-1).

Circulation of Cerebrospinal Fluid

The flow of fluid through the ventricular system is determined by the anatomy. The only way out of the ventricles is through the foramina of Magendie and Luschka. From the cisterna magna, the CSF moves into all parts of the subarachnoid space. The general direction of movement is around the cerebral hemispheres and cerebellum towards the dural venous sinuses. Movement into and out of the spinal subarachnoid space is slower, but too rapid to be explained by diffusion. Tracers introduced into the CSF move in both directions between the lumbar cistern and the cisterna magna, although caudally directed flow predominates. It is widely believed that turbulence is generated in the CSF by the pulsation of arteries.

Absorption of Cerebrospinal Fluid

The sites of absorption of the CSF into the blood were discovered in 1914 by Lewis H. Weed (1886–1952), an American anatomist. His principal method was the tracing of colored and particulate substances introduced into the CSF. The findings have been repeatedly confirmed and amplified by the use of modern methods.

Most of the CSF passes into the venous blood of the dural sinuses. Absorption is through **arachnoid villi.** These are microscopic protrusions of thin arachnoid membrane through holes in the dura (see Chap. 28, Fig. 28-2).

Each arachnoid villus behaves as a tiny valve. When the pressure of the CSF is higher than that of the blood in the sinus, the fluid flows into the blood. On occasions when the venous pressure is higher, blood cannot pass in the opposite direction to enter the subarachnoid space. The mechanism of the val-

Table 30-1. Comparison of Plasma with Cerebrospinal Fluid

Solute	Concentration (approximate)	
	Blood Plasma	*Cerebrospinal Fluid*
Sodium	140 mM	145 mM
Potassium	5 mM	2 mM
Chloride	10 mM	130 mM
Protein	7 grams per liter	0.2 grams per liter
	(55% albumin, 40% globulin, 5% fibrinogen)	(90% albumin, 10% globulin, no fibrinogen)

vular action is not fully understood. It is possible that the CSF passes through holes in or between the arachnoid cells when the villus is distended by the pressure of the CSF. A higher pressure in the venous sinus would allow the intercellular spaces to close and would also close the lumen of the villus by pressing it flat. Electron microscopy reveals tight junctions between arachnoid cells. There are, however, great numbers of vesicles in the cytoplasm, and the vesicles take up tracers introduced into the CSF. Vesicular transport is therefore a mechanism for absorption of at least some of the CSF into the blood.

Arachnoid villi are most numerous around the superior sagittal sinus, where aggregations of the structures from **arachnoid granulations** or Pacchionian bodies (named after the Italian anatomist Antonio Pacchioni, 1665–1726). Arachnoid granulations, which are easily seen with the unaided eye, become larger with age and often produce identations of the internal surfaces of the parietal bones. Structures identical to the cranial arachnoid villi are associated with veins that leave the spinal canal through the intervertebral foramina. Where each vein pierces the dura, a tuft of arachnoid villi protrudes into the lumen. A small proportion of the CSF leaves the subarachnoid space by diffusing into peripheral nerves. The arachnoid is continuous with the perineurium, so some CSF enters the endoneurial connective tissue and is absorbed into blood and lymphatic vessels.

Functions of the Cerebrospinal Fluid

The most obvious function of the CSF is protection of the brain from impact with the bony cranium. The CSF also serves to carry away products of metabolism, including water and carbon dioxide. In conjunction with the blood–brain barrier, the CSF provides an extracellular fluid appropriate for the nutrition of neurons and neuroglia.

Clinical Significance of Cerebrospinal Fluid

Raised Intracranial Pressure

The symptoms and signs of a space-occupying intracranial lesion or of generalized swelling of the brain (cerebral edema) are:

1. *Headache,* typically throbbing, due to pressure of the brain and of arteries upon the dura
2. *Vomiting,* which is often sudden. The causative mechanism is not fully understood
3. *Slowing of heart and respiration,* attributed to pressure on the medulla
4. *Stupor,* proceeding to coma, attributed to compression of the midbrain
5. *False localizing signs,* such as those of upper motor neuron paresis, or palsies of cranial nerves III or VI, are attributed to pressure upon or around the brain stem
6. *Papilledema*

Papilledema

Abnormally high intracranial pressure is transmitted through the tenuous subarachnoid space of the optic nerve to the optic disc, where the axons from the retina leave the eye. The disc (*papilla*) becomes swollen (*edema*tous), and this change can be seen with an ophthalmoscope. The swelling is due partly to excess extracellular fluid and partly to dilatation of the optic axons, in which axoplasmic transport has been partially dammed by the pressure within the dural sheath of the optic nerve. The raised pressure also compresses the tributaries of the central retinal vein, so that the optic disc is surrounded by dilated veins. The term "choked discs" is a synonym for papilledema.

Papilledema is usually due to *raised intracranial pressure,* but it is also seen in very severe *arterial hypertension* in conjunction with other retinal abnormalities. Unilateral papilledema can be due to *thrombosis of the central retinal vein* or to *retrobulbar neuritis*. The latter condition is inflammation in the optic nerve around a demyelinating lesion of multiple sclerosis.

For reasons explained in Chapter 28, lumbar puncture should not be undertaken in the presence of papilledema.

Hydrocephalus

An abnormally large volume of cerebrospinal fluid accumulates if there is an obstruction to its circulation or absorption. **Hydrocephalus** (from the Greek words for "water" and "head") is **internal** if the CSF cannot escape from part or all of the ventricular system. Some of the classical experiments described earlier in this chapter produced internal hydrocephalus. The most common causes of hydrocephalus in children are stenosis (abnormal narrowness) of the cerebral aqueduct and a malformation of the medulla, the cerebellum, and the occipital bone that obstructs the foramina of the fourth ventricle. The latter malformation is usually associated with a spinal meningomyelocele (see Chap. 5).

As hydrocephalus develops, the infant's head swells and there is destruction of cerebral tissue around the expanding ventricles. Cerebral cortical function is often spared, despite considerable thinning of the walls of the lateral ventricles. Hydrocephalus is treated by inserting a tube containing a valve to shunt CSF from a lateral ventricle into a vein.

In older children and adults, hydrocephalus may be due to any disease that intereferes with the flow of CSF. For example, bacterial meningitis can lead to scars that obstruct the apertures in the roof of the fourth ventricle, or a tumor may impede flow through the third ventricle. The head cannot expand after it has stopped growing, so the enlarging ventricles compress and destroy brain tissue, especially the white matter of the cerebral hemispheres. **Communicating hydrocephalus** is due to ob-

struction outside the ventricular system. For example, the arachnoid villi can be blocked by pus or blood after meningitis or a subarachnoid hemorrhage. All four ventricles become enlarged if the obstruction does not clear spontaneously. Enlargement of the ventricles and the subarachnoid space is also seen when there is considerable atrophy of the brain, such as the cortical degeneration of advanced Alzheimer's disease (see Chap. 25).

Collection of Cerebrospinal Fluid

Unless contraindicated (papilledema), collection of CSF for diagnostic purposes is done by **lumbar puncture** (spinal tap). With local anesthesia, a needle made for the purpose is inserted in the midline, halfway between the dorsal spines of vertebrae L3 and L4 or L4 and L5, with the patient lying curled up and on one side. There is no risk of injuring the spinal cord. The nerve roots forming the cauda equina are harmlessly pushed aside by the needle. The pressure is measured as the vertical height of a column of CSF in a glass tube connected to the needle (normally 50 to 200 mm of CSF), and there is normally a brisk rise in pressure if the veins of the neck are compressed. No more than 5 ml of CSF is collected. The patient has a headache, exacerbated (made worse) by movement, for some hours afterwards. The headache is caused by the brain bumping against the sensitive dura.

The specimen is examined for the presence of cells (especially leukocytes), plasma proteins, and bacteria. Special tests are available for some individual diseases.

Tanycytes and Neurons That Contact the Cerebrospinal Fluid

Most of the lining of the ventricular system consists of ordinary ependyma, but in a few places in the third and fourth ventricles there are **tanycytes** (see Chap. 2). Those in the floor of the third ventricle are the only ones about which much is known. These cells have boutonlike endings on hypothalamic neurons and on the blood vessels of the median eminence. Anatomically they are ideally sited to detect chemical agents such as hormones in the CSF, and to respond by secreting substances that modify the activities of hypothalamic neurons and adenohypophysial cells (see Chap. 26).

In many animals, neuronal processes have been seen with the electron microscope to protrude between ependymal cells into the CSF. Such neurons are most numerous in the dorsal part of the hypothalamus. There are even neurons with their cell-bodies and many processes lying on the surface of the ependyma of the third ventricle. Such cells are conspicuous, but not numerous, in scanning electron micrographs of the ependymal surface. Nothing is known of the functions of CSF-contacting neurons.

The **subcommissural organ** is a conspicuous area of atypical ependyma in the dorsal wall of the cerebral aqueduct, ventral to the posterior commissure. It is present in all vertebrate animals. The tall ependymocytes contain granules of a glycoprotein, which is secreted into the CSF. In some animals (including fetal, but not adult human beings) the secretion from the subcommissural organ solidifies to form a long string known as **Reissner's fiber.** Ernst Reissner (1824–1878) was a German anatomist. The fiber, surrounded by CSF, continues through the aqueduct, the fourth ventricle, and the central canal to the caudal end of the spinal cord.

Circumventricular Organs

Five small regions beneath the ependyma of the third and fourth ventricle have atypical blood vessels. The capillaries are permeable to proteins and are surrounded by extracellular spaces. Elsewhere in the central nervous system the capillary blood vessels are impermeable and very little extracellular space is seen in conventional electron micrographs (though there may be more in the living state). In the circumventricular organs large molecules can move freely between the blood and the nervous tissue.

The **neurohypophysis** is the largest circumventricular organ. It has numerous endocrine functions. The **epiphysis** or pineal gland is the second largest circumventricular organ.

The **subfornical organ,** also known as the intercolumnar tubercle, is in the roof of the third ventricle. In animals, the subfornical organ, which projects to the hypothalamus, responds to increased circulating levels of angiotensin and stimulates drinking. The human subfornical organ may have an equivalent function. Another circumventricular organ of the third ventricle is in the lamina terminalis, dorsal to the optic chiasma. This is the *organon vasculosum laminae terminalis* (**OVLT**); it has also been called the "supraoptic crest." The OVLT may mediate feedback of the endocrine system upon the hypothalamus.

The **area postrema** is in the floor of the fourth ventricle, at the caudalmost level of the "open" medulla. It is called a "chemoreceptor trigger zone" because in animals it detects toxic substances, notably the emetic drug *apomorphine.* Vomiting caused by such substances is initiated by connections of the area postrema with the underlying reticular formation, the solitary nucleus, and the dorsal nucleus of the vagus nerve. The function of the area postrema may be to induce the vomiting of incompletely absorbed swallowed poisons.

Index

Page numbers in *italics* refer to entries in figures or tables; often the same page contains relevant text as well. **Bold face** indicates a definition, a biographical note, or the principal treatment of a subject in the text.